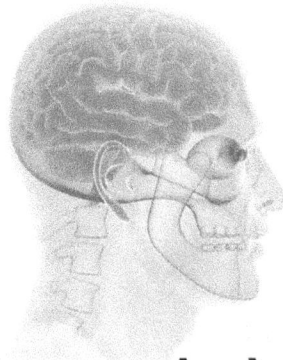

Emergencies in Neuro-Ophthalmology

A Case Based Approach

Emergencies in Neuro-Ophthalmology

A Case Based Approach

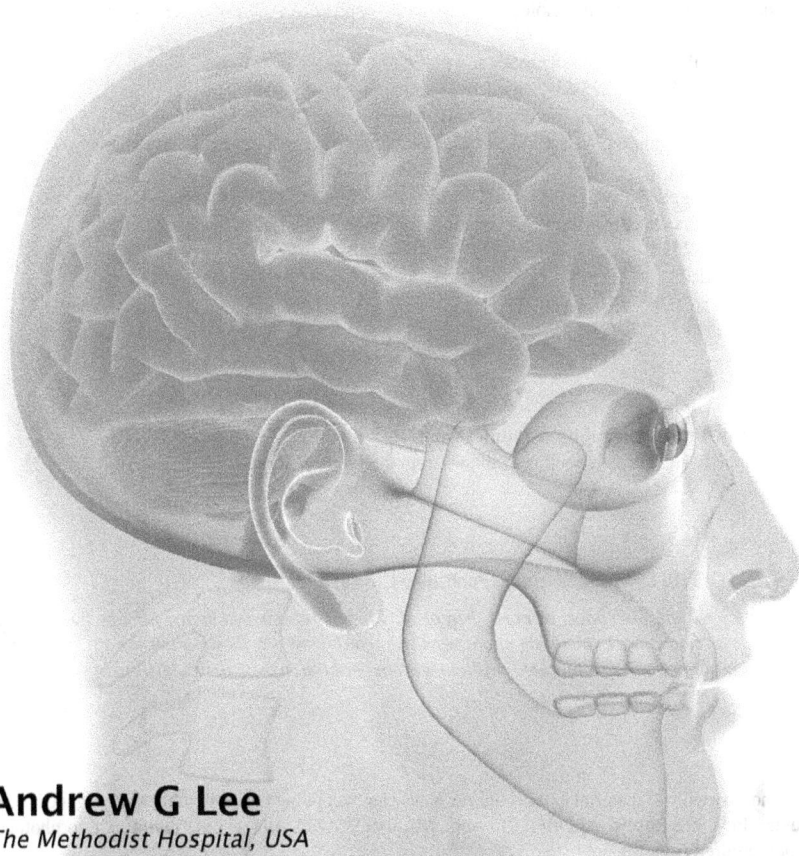

Andrew G Lee
The Methodist Hospital, USA

Paul W Brazis
Mayo Clinic, USA

Mansoor Mughal & **Fabiana Policeni**
University of Iowa Hospitals and Clinics, USA

World Scientific

NEW JERSEY · LONDON · SINGAPORE · BEIJING · SHANGHAI · HONG KONG · TAIPEI · CHENNAI

Published by

World Scientific Publishing Co. Pte. Ltd.

5 Toh Tuck Link, Singapore 596224

USA office: 27 Warren Street, Suite 401-402, Hackensack, NJ 07601

UK office: 57 Shelton Street, Covent Garden, London WC2H 9HE

Library of Congress Cataloging-in-Publication Data
Emergencies in neuro-ophthalmology : a case based approach / Andrew G. Lee . [et al.].
      p. ; cm.
      Includes bibliographical references and index.
      ISBN-13: 978-981-4295-01-7 (hardcover : alk. paper)
      ISBN-10: 981-4295-01-9 (hardcover : alk. paper)
      1. Neuroophthalmology--Case studies. 2. Ophthalmologic emergencies--Case studies.
I. Lee, Andrew G.
      [DNLM: 1. Optic Nerve Diseases--diagnosis--Case Reports. 2. Emergencies--Case Reports.
3.   Optic Nerve Diseases--therapy--Case Reports. WW 280 E53 2010]
      RE725.E44 2010
      617.7'32--dc22

      2010011911

British Library Cataloguing-in-Publication Data
A catalogue record for this book is available from the British Library.

Typeset by Stallion Press
Email: enquiries@stallionpress.com

Dedication

Drs. Lee and Brazis would like to dedicate this volume to
Dr. Neil R. Miller, their teacher, friend, and source of inspiration.

About the Authors

Andrew G. Lee MD is currently the Chairman of The Methodist Hospital (TMH) Department of Ophthalmology, and a Professor of Ophthalmology, Neurology and Neurosurgery, Weill Cornell Medical College. He is an Adjunct Professor of Ophthalmology at the University of Iowa Hospitals and Clinics, and a Clinical Professor of Ophthalmology, UTMB Galveston.

Paul W. Brazis MD is Professor of Ophthalmology and Neurology at the Mayo Clinic, Jacksonville, Florida.

At the time of this publication, Mansoor Moghul MD and Fabiana Policeni MD were fellows in Neuro-ophthalmology at the University of Iowa Hospitals and Clinics.

Preface

The management of emergent neuro-ophthalmic conditions can be a life saving encounter for the general ophthalmologist. This book is designed to help the comprehensive ophthalmologist to make emergency triage decisions for initial evaluation and treatment of potentially vision- or life-threatening conditions. This text is case-based and is intended to provide the reader with the opinion and expertise of two neuro-ophthalmologists. One, Dr. Lee is an ophthalmology-based neuro-ophthalmologist and the other, Dr. Brazis is a neurology-based neuro-ophthalmologist. Dr. Moghul and Dr. Policeni collected and collated the case vignettes during their fellowship with Dr. Lee at the University of Iowa Hospitals and Clinics.

It is the goal of this text to provide a concise, easy to read, and practical guide to the emergent evaluation of these neuro-ophthalmic conditions. This book is designed to be a quick read and not to be all inclusive or comprehensive. The reader is directed to longer and more comprehensive neuro-ophthalmic texts for this information. It is also not our intention to provide anatomy, pharmacology, physiology, or other basic mechanisms of disease. Instead, this text is meant to be a quick reference and resource for the clinician in the emergency room or in the clinic facing a potentially vision- or life-threatening emergency and to provide immediate guidance for potentially "high stakes" decision making. We also wish to emphasize that the recommendations of this text represent the authors' own opinions on management and are not intended to be, nor should they be, construed as a "standard of care." The case vignettes are based upon real clinical cases but the clinical details of each case have been modified for teaching purposes and represent composite rather than individual histories.

Each case vignette is composed of the relevant and concise medical history; the neuro-ophthalmic exam findings; the clinical and exam findings with demonstrative figures; and finally the expert opinion for management provided by Dr. Lee and Dr. Brazis.

We hope that the reader will enjoy the format and content of this text and we invite comments and feedback on the utility of our work.

Andrew G. Lee MD
Paul W. Brazis MD

Acknowledgments

Dr. Lee would like to recognize and to thank his patient and always loving wife, Hilary A. Beaver MD for putting up with the writing of textbook #5. As the saying goes, "No man succeeds without a good woman behind him" and in my case I have had the honor of having five supportive women in my life; one wife (Hilary), my mother (Rosalind Lee MD), two daughters (Rachael and Virginia) and a sister (Amy Lee Wirts MD), so I feel blessed times five. I also thank my father (Alberto C. Lee MD) for instilling in me a passion for medicine and my brother (Richard Lee) for being a source of real world wisdom and providing a reality check from the non-MD side of the family. Finally, Dr. Lee thanks Dr. Brazis his co-editor for being the best friend and neuro-ophthalmology buddy a guy could ask for.

Dr. Brazis would like to thank his family, especially his wife Elizabeth, for their support and love. He also thanks Dr. Andrew Lee, his friend and colleague, who has taught him much over the years in neuro-ophthalmology, but also concerning friendship and life in general.

Contents

1A

Acute Painful Ptosis, Complete Ophthalmoplegia with a Red Eye

CASE NO. 1A

A 55-year-old white female presented in the emergency room (ER) with a chief complaint of the onset of a headache during the previous four days. The headache resolved the following day, but she began having swelling of her right eye (OD). This worsened over the following few days and she developed diplopia. She related no eye pain but did complain that the right side of her face was numb.

On examination, her visual acuity was 20/100 OD and 20/20 OS. The pupillary examination showed a dilated and fixed pupil OD; the pupil OS was normally reactive to light. Ocular motility showed complete ophthalmoplegia OD and was full OS (Fig. 1A.1). External examination showed complete ptosis and marked proptosis OD (Fig. 1A.2). Hertel measurement showed 7 mm of proptosis OD. There was a prominent orbital bruit over the right eye. Slit lamp examination showed dilatation of the conjunctiva and episcleral vessels with diffuse injection. There was no chemosis. The cornea was clear, the anterior chamber was quiet, and the lens was normal. Examination OS was unremarkable. Intraocular pressure was 26 mm Hg OD and 18 mm Hg OS. Ophthalmoscopic examination was normal in each eye.

Discussion

Dr. Brazis' comments: The above clinical scenario is most consistent with a carotid-cavernous sinus fistula (CCF) which is an abnormal

1

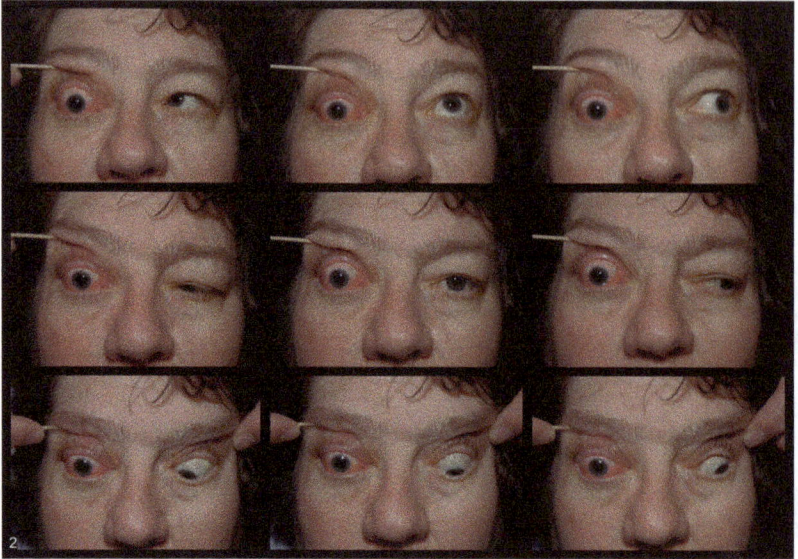

Fig. 1A.1. Ocular motility photography showing the almost complete ophthalmoplegia in the right eye.

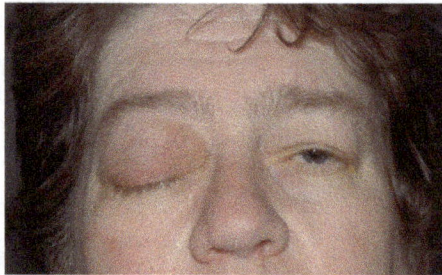

Fig. 1A.2. External photography showing the complete right ptosis.

communication between the cavernous sinus and the carotid arterial system. CCFs can be classified by etiology (e.g. traumatic versus spontaneous), by velocity of blood flow (e.g. high versus low flow), or by anatomy (e.g. direct versus dural; internal carotid artery versus external carotid artery supply versus both). In this patient, I would be concerned about a direct high flow connection between the cavernous segment of the internal carotid artery and the cavernous sinus. These fistulas are of a high flow type, and because they are often caused by a single tear in the arterial wall they are thus called direct CCFs.

Direct CCFs represent 70% to 90% of all CCFs in most large clinical series. They occur in both men and women and may occur at any age. A direct CCF results from a single tear in the wall of the cavernous segment of the internal carotid artery. This produces a direct connection between the artery and one or more of the venous channels within the cavernous sinus. Direct CCFs most often are the result of head trauma, especially motor vehicle accidents, fights, and falls. The injury may be extremely severe or quite trivial. A substantial minority of direct CCFs are caused by rupture of a pre-existing aneurysm of the cavernous segment of the internal carotid artery. Direct CCFs may also be the iatrogenic, occurring after various diagnostic and therapeutic procedures (e.g. carotid endarterectomy, cranial and percutaneous retro-Gasserian procedure for the trigeminal neuralgia, transphenoidal surgery, or maxillofacial surgeries).

Although direct CCFs are usually not thought to be life-threatening, there are numerous reports of patients experiencing significant and even fatal epistaxis, subarachnoid hemorrhage, or intracerebral hemorrhage from rupture of the fistula. The ocular manifestations of a direct CCF are usually ipsilateral to the side of the fistula but may be bilateral or even contralateral. The lateralization of ocular manifestations depends on the venous drainage of the cavernous sinuses, including the connections between the two sinuses through the intercavernous sinuses and the basilar sinus, the presence or absence of cortical venous drainage, and the presence or absence of thrombosis within the sinus or a superior ophthalmic vein on one or both sides.

Proptosis is a common sign, occurring in almost all patients. In most cases proptosis develops rapidly on the side of the fistula and becomes pronounced within a few days. In the early stages of a direct CCF, the eyelids may become moderately or severely swollen. When the superior ophthalmic vein is enlarged, the medial portion of the upper eyelid may be ptotic or swollen. Conjunctival chemosis to some degree occurs in most patients. In more severe cases, the inferior palpebral conjunctiva may prolapse through the interpalpebral fissure and rarely may cause conjunctival necrosis or superinfection. As arterial blood is forced anteriorly into the orbital veins, the conjunctival and episcleral veins becomes dilated, tortuous, and filled with arterial blood. This "arterialization" of the conjunctival vessels is the hallmark of a CCF. Although it may initially be mistaken for conjunctivitis or episcleritis, the dilation and tortuosity of the affected vessels is usually quite distinctive, running to the limbus and often arching back in a loop. Ocular pulsations are caused by transmission of the pulse waves from the internal carotid or ophthalmic artery to the ophthalmic veins. Abnormal ocular pulsations may be visible on applanation or other tonometry and may sometimes produce pulsating exophthalmos that may be palpalble.

Exposure keratopathy is the most frequent corneal sign encountered in patients with a direct CCF. The keratopathy may be aggravated by a concomitant trigeminal neuropathy caused by injury or by the effects of the fistula on the trigeminal nerve within the cavernous sinus. In some patients with a direct CCF, the initial symptom may be a pulsatile tinnitus or subjective bruit which may or may not be associated with an audible bruit. Diplopia occurs in 60% to 70% of patients with direct CCF. The diplopia may be caused by dysfunction of one or more of the ocular motor nerves, the extraocular muscles, or both, and the degree of motility limitation varies from mild to complete ophthalmoplegia. Visual loss associated with a direct CCF may be immediate or delayed. Immediate visual loss is usually caused by ocular or optic nerve damage at the time of the head injury. Delayed visual loss is usually caused by retinal dysfunction, but it may be related to vitreous hemorrhage, central retinal vein occlusion, angle closure glaucoma from anterior rotation of the ciliary body, anterior ischemic optic neuropathy, or even corneal ulceration. Dilation of the retinal veins may be seen and can be asymptomatic but can produce venous stasis retinopathy or even frank central retinal vein occlusion with macular edema and diffuse retinal hemorrhages.

Occasionally, patients complain of facial pain in the distribution of the first and rarely the second division of the trigeminal nerve. Some patients will have decreased corneal sensation, decreased facial sensation, or both, perhaps related to ischemia or compression of the ophthalmic or maxillary divisions of the trigeminal nerve within the cavernous sinus. Glaucoma may develop in up to 30% to 50% of patients, and most commonly the rise in intraocular pressure is due to increased episcleral venous pressure or orbital congestion. Neovascular glaucoma may also occur associated with chronic retinal hypoxia and retinal neovascularization.

Finally, as in this patient, a direct CCF should be suspected in any patient who suddenly develops chemosis, proptosis, and a red eye. If there is no history of trauma, one should consider the possibility of a ruptured cavernous aneurysm.

Dr. Lee's comments: Dr. Brazis has provided a nice summary of direct and indirect CCFs. The indirect CCF may spontaneously involute and in the absence of vision threatening proptosis, exposure keratopathy, debilitating ophthalmoplegia, visual loss, or severe pain, many patients can be observed for spontaneous resolution from the natural history of thrombosis in these lesions. Non-catheter based neuroimaging (e.g. MRI and MRA or CTA) might be sufficient to confirm the diagnosis but most patients require catheter angiography. We have also used orbital ultrasound to follow the patient for spontaneous thrombosis and determine if clinical worsening might be paradoxically related to radiographic thrombosis and not an increase in the flow in the CCF. Halback *et al.* reviewed the angiographic and clinical data from 155 patients with CCF. The features associated with an increased risk of morbidity and mortality included the following:

- presence of a pseudoaneurysm
- large varix of the cavernous sinus
- venous drainage to cortical veins, and
- thrombosis of venous outflow pathways distant from the fistula.

The clinical signs and symptoms of a potentially "hazardous" CCFs included:

- increased intracranial pressure
- rapidly progressive proptosis
- diminished visual acuity
- hemorrhage and
- transient ischemic attacks.

The cortical venous drainage from the carotid cavernous fistula is due to occlusion or absence of the normal venous outflow pathways and can produce increased intracranial pressure or intraparenchymal hemorrhage. Cavernous sinus varix and extension into the subarachnoid space (with associated risk of potentially fatal subarachnoid hemorrhage) are also considered to be angiographic risk factors for morbidity and mortality. Standard catheter angiography in these patients might be diagnostic, prognostic, and in some cases therapeutic (i.e. angiographically induced thrombosis of the CCF). Direct CCF, on the other hand, typically require catheter angiography as the clinical signs and symptoms are more acute and severe, and as Dr. Brazis mentioned, the catheter angiogram can be diagnostic and in the same or sequential sittings be coupled with endovascular treatment of the CCF.

CT scanning, CT angiography (CTA), MR imaging, and MR angiography (MRA) can be used to confirm the diagnosis, showing enlargement of the extraocular muscles, dilation of one or both superior ophthalmic veins, enlargement of the affected cavernous sinus, and abnormal intracranial vessels (e.g. enlarged or increased flow voids on MRA or MRI in cavernous sinus). The ultimate diagnostic test, however, is catheter angiography.

Contrast brain MRI in this patient demonstrated right proptosis, enlarged flow void inside the right cavernous sinus, and an enlarged superior ophthalmic vein (Figs. 1A.3 and 1A.4). Catheter angiography revealed an internal carotid artery aneurysm (Fig. 1A.5) as the cause of the CCF.

The optimum treatment of a direct CCF is closure of the abnormal arteriovenous communication with preservation of the internal

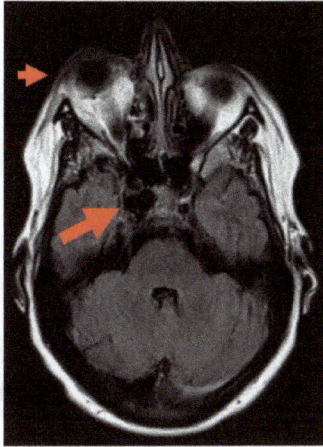

Fig. 1A.3. Brain MRI axial T1 without contrast demonstrates right proptosis (*small arrow*) and enlarged flow void inside the right cavernous sinus (*large arrow*).

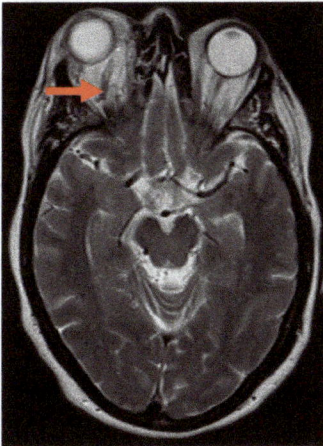

Fig. 1A.4. Brain MRI Axial T2 demonstrates the enlargement of the right superior ophthalmic vein (*arrow*).

carotid artery patency. Endovascular closure of direct CCF is most often accompanied by embolization using a variety of agents, primarily coils and detachable balloons. Complications most often result from balloon occlusion of a direct CCF when there is planned or

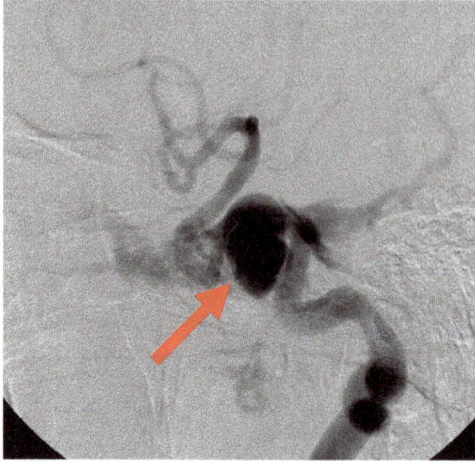

Fig. 1A.5. Right carotid angiogram demonstrates an aneurysm in the internal carotid artery (*arrow*).

unplanned occlusion of the internal carotid artery. These complications, primarily those related to reduction or interruption of the blood supply to the ipsilateral eye and cerebral hemisphere, include stroke and even death. Once the fistula is successfully closed, most of the ocular symptoms and signs resolve or will at least improve and do not recur. Of all the symptoms and signs of a direct CCF, visual loss is least likely to improve after successful treatment even when the internal carotid artery remains patent.

1B

Chronic Painless Ptosis, Complete Ophthalmoplegia with a Red Eye

CASE NO. 1B

A 69-year-old man presented with a 12-week history of a red eye OS which was initially felt to be "conjunctivitis" by an outside eye doctor and was treated with topical antibiotics for two weeks, then with topical antihistamines for two weeks, following which topical antivirals were added, and finally topical steroids without improvement. His symptoms worsened and he developed double vision which was worse on upgaze. He also noticed a "whooshing" sound in his ears, more noticeable just before going to sleep. He denied any periocular pain, headache, or visual blurring. There was no history of trauma as well as no history of thyroid eye disease, and he did not smoke cigarettes. The remainder of his medical history was non-contributory.

On examination, visual acuity was 20/20 OU. There was no relative afferent pupillary defect or anisocoria. There was 2 mm of ptosis in the left upper lid (Fig. 1B.1) and mild to moderate lid edema OS. Slit lamp examination showed diffuse subconjunctival hemorrhage OS with dilated and tortuous episcleral and conjunctival vessels extending to the limbus and looping back (Fig. 1B.2). The intraocular pressure (IOP) was 12 mm Hg OD and 28 mm Hg OS. Optic disc examination showed a cup-to-disc ratio of 0.3 OU and the remainder of the fundus exam was normal. Hertel measurement showed mild proptosis OS of 2 mm. Goldmann perimetry and OCT were normal OU. The left eye had a –2 underaction of elevation with a 15 prism diopter left hypotropia in upgaze.

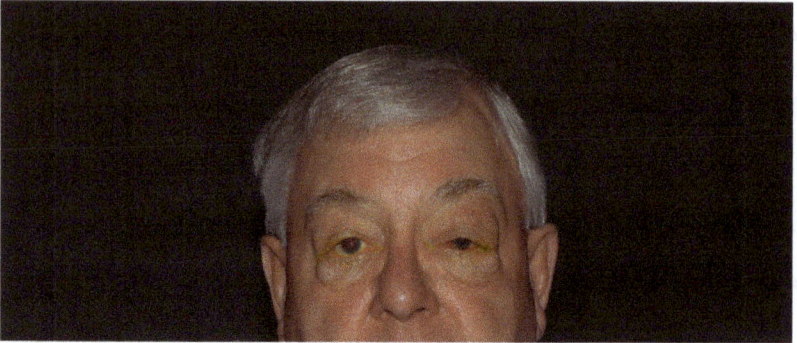

Fig. 1B.1. External photograph showing a left ptosis.

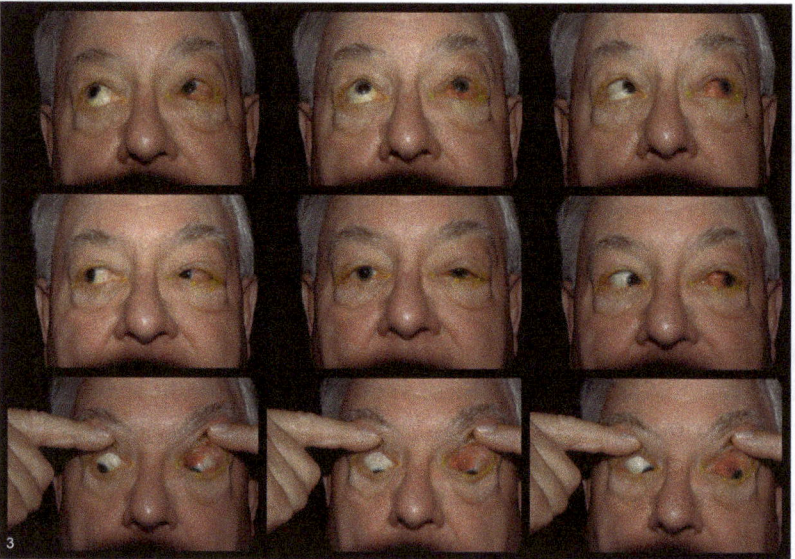

Fig. 1B.2. The left eye had a –2 underaction of elevation with a 15 prism diopter left hypotropia in upgaze. The left eye showed a left diffuse subconjunctival hemorrhage with tortuous vessels suggestive of "arterialization" of the episcleral vessels.

Dr. Lee. In a patient with a chronic "red eye" unresponsive to multiple different topical therapies, the general ophthalmologist should consider alternative etiologies to the typical "red eye" list. In light of this patient's additional symptoms (e.g. diplopia, ptosis, and proptosis), the clinical localization of the problem shifts from the anterior segment to the orbit. The distinctive clinical sign here is the "arterialization" of the conjunctival and episcleral vessels (Fig. 1B.2), with the classic dilated and tortuous vessels extending to and from the limbus. Interestingly, the intervening conjunctiva is often white, also giving the clinician a clue that the etiology is not a typical allergic, inflammatory, or infectious "conjunctivitis." The additional symptom of a subjective bruit in this case suggests a vascular etiology and the next most appropriate step is imaging. Elevated IOP and secondary glaucoma can occur due to orbital congestion or increased episcleral venous pressure. Rarely, patients may have angle closure from anterior rotation of a swollen ciliary body. Treating the IOP with glaucoma drops may be useful as a temporizing measure but the underlying etiology needs to be identified and treated. I would consider CCF to be the leading clinical diagnosis in a case like this one. The applanation tonometry mires sometimes give a clue to an increased pulse pressure in the measurement of the IOP. Orbital ultrasound might show a dilated superior ophthalmic vein and arterialization of flow can be obtained using orbital Doppler flow studies. CT scan or MR scan typically shows the dilated superior ophthalmic vein and might show enlargement or even flow voids in the cavernous sinus. Clinical or radiographic evidence for cortical venous drainage should be sought and might be an indication for more aggressive treatment for a carotid cavernous fistula.

Dr. Brazis. The above clinical scenario is most consistent with a CCF. The differentiating features for direct and high flow versus indirect and slow flow fistula have been discussed previously.

Course. Cranial MRI/MRA (Fig. 1B.3) showed a dilated left superior ophthalmic vein with arterialized flow. There was no clinical or radiographic evidence for cortical venous drainage. The patient was observed initially but continued to worsen and underwent a diagnostic catheter angiogram that confirmed the diagnosis of an indirect CCF with internal carotid artery feeders and this was followed by

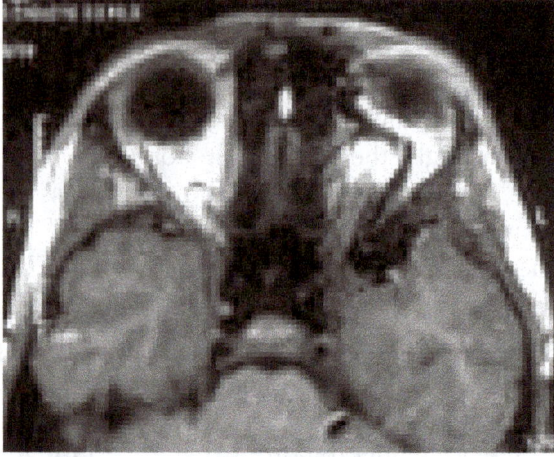

Fig. 1B.3. MRI shows dilated left superior ophthalmic vein.

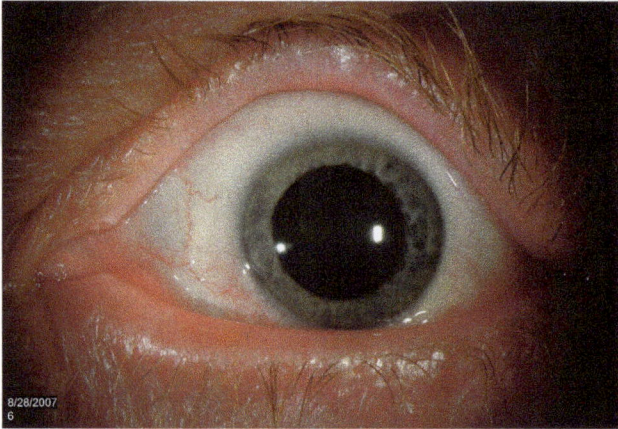

Fig. 1B.4. Color photograph of the left eye (after dilation) following successful obliteration of the CCF, and with endovascular coiling procedure shows marked resolution of the arterialization of the conjunctival and episcleral vessels.

endovascular closure of the fistula. The subjective bruit immediately resolved after the procedure and over the next two months the ptosis, lid edema, proptosis, ophthalmoplegia, and red eye all completely resolved (Fig. 1B.4).

REFERENCES

Barrow DL, Spector RH, Braun IF, *et al.* (1985) Classification and treatment of spontaneous carotid-cavernous sinus fistulas. *J Neurosurg* **62**:248–256.

Debrun GM, Vinuela F, Fox AJ, *et al.* (1988) Indications for treatment and classification of 132 carotid-cavernous fistulas. *Neurosurgery* **22**:285–289.

Halbach VV, Hieshima GB, Higashida TT, Reicher M. (1987) Carotid cavernous fistulae: Indications for urgent treatment. *Am J Roentgenology* **149**:587–593.

Taki W, Nakahara I, Nishi S, *et al.* (1994) Pathogenesis and therapeutic considerations of carotid-cavernous sinus fistulas. *Acta Neurochir* **127**:6–14.

2A

Acute Painless Homonymous Hemianopsia

CASE NO. 2A

A 67-year-old woman presented in the emergency room complaining of grayish cloud over her right side vision which started in the morning. She also related some imbalance of walking that she felt was due to her visual field defect. When the symptoms did not resolve after about an hour, she decided to seek medical attention. Past medical history was significant for hypertension and diabetes. She was on oral antihypertensive and diabetic treatments. She did not smoke or drink. She had no prior ocular history. She denied any other neurologic signs or symptoms. There was no headadche, jaw claudication, or temporal artery tenderness.

On examination, the patient's visual acuity was 20/25 in each eye. External examination was unremarkable and the temporal arteries were normal. Ocular motility was full in both eyes. The Goldmann visual field (Fig. 2A.1) revealed a dense right homonymous hemianopia. Slit lamp examination was normal. Ophthalmoscopy was unremarkable in both eyes.

Discussion

Dr. Brazis. A complete right homonymous hemianopia in this case indicates damage to retrochiasmal pathways on the left side. Because the hemianopia is complete, localization to specific structures (e.g. optic tract, occipital lobe, etc.,) cannot be determined without

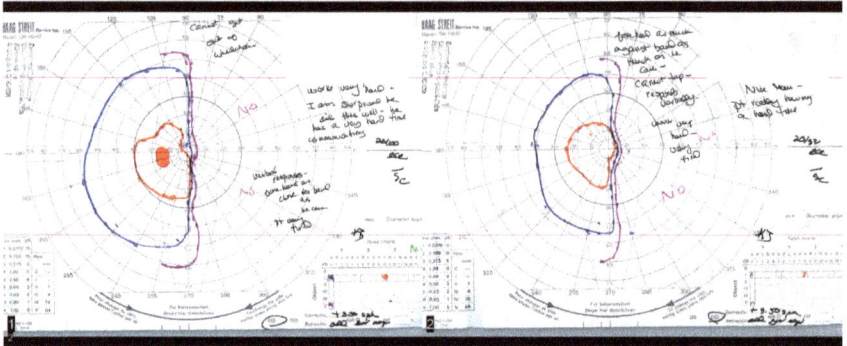

Fig. 2A.1. Goldman visual field showing the complete right homonymous hemianopia.

neuroimaging. However, an acute homonymous hemianopia without other neurologic impairments suggests an occipital lesion. As the onset of the visual field loss was acute, a vascular event, e.g. an ischemic infarct or cerebral hemorrhage, is the most likely etiology for the visual field defect.

The patient needs urgent neuroimaging. If an intracerebral hemorrhage is discovered, there may be little else to offer except supportive care and possible admission to the hospital. However, if the deficit is due to an acute ischemic infarction and the patient otherwise satisfies the criteria for treatment with tissue plasminogen activator (tPA), a tPA injection would be a consideration as long as the patient and/or her family fully understand and are willing to accept the potential risk of intracerebral hemorrhage (approximately 6.4% of patients injected) with this treatment.

Inclusion criteria for tPA treatment include:

- A clear time of onset of symptoms
- Injection within 3 hours onset of symptoms (defined as last time patient was symptom-free) – remember "Time is Brain"
- Measurable deficit on the NIH stroke scale (NIHSS)
- Patient's age >18 years

Exclusion criteria for tPA treatment include:

- Intracranial hemorrhage or early changes of major infarction on CT scan
- History of stroke or head trauma in last 3 months
- Major surgery within last 14 days
- History of intracranial hemorrhage
- Severe hypertension (BP >185/110 mm Hg)
- Rapidly improving or minor symptoms
- Symptoms suggestive of subarachnoid hemorrhage
- Gastrointestinal or urinary tract hemorrhage within last 21 days
- Arterial puncture at non-compressible site within last 7 days
- Seizure at onset of stroke
- Use of oral anticoagulants or heparin
- Recent myocardial infarction
- Protime (PT) >15 seconds
- Platelet count <100,000/mm
- Glucose <50 or >400 mg/dl

The patient needs to have urgent neuroimaging in order to consider tPA treatment. We perform CT imaging including dynamic CT scanning with CT angiography and CT perfusion studies that rely on rapid rate scanning to follow the passage of an intravenously injected iodinated contrast agent through the cerebral circulation. Reduced cerebral perfusion in the absence of a cerebral blood volume abnormality is indicative of ischemic, yet potentially salvageable, brain tissue. Mismatch can thus be obtained by comparing the size of the cerebral blood volume abnormality with that of the perfusion disturbance. A mismatch implies tissue is at risk.

In this patient, a CT scan revealed no cerebral hemorrhage but the CT perfusion study (Fig. 2A.2) revealed an area of left occipital ischemia. Therefore, intravenous infusion of tPA would be warranted to attempt to improve her visual field deficit. Patients with cerebral infarct who received tPA are at least 30% more likely to have

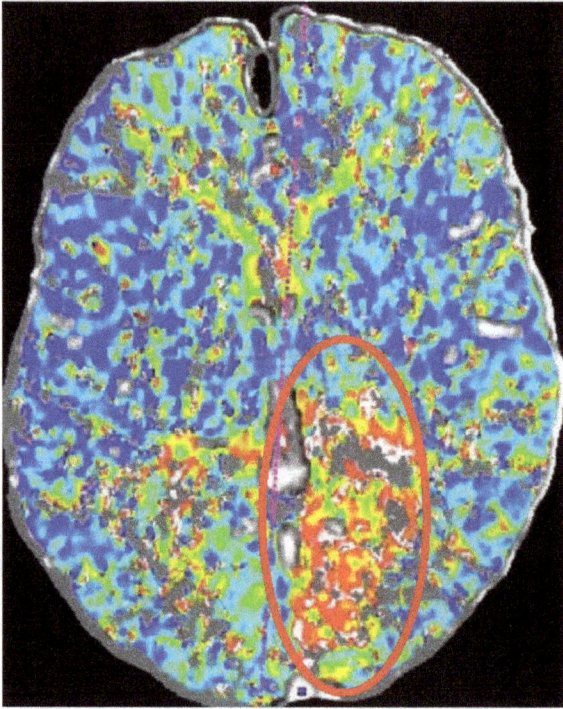

Fig. 2A.2. CT perfusion of the brain demonstrates increased mean transient time in the left PCA distribution consistent with ischemic change (circle).

minimal neurologic or no disability at 3 months as compared with patient's who do not receive this drug. Thirty-one to fifty percent have complete or near-complete recovery at one year versus 20%–38% of a placebo group.

Treating physician should document in the medical record the reasons for the use or non-use of thrombolytic drugs. If the patient meets the treatment guidelines, and the ophthalmologist and the patient/family choose not to use thrombolysis, then we strongly recommend that the rationale and the clear discussion of the benefits and risks be documented. Likewise, if the patient does not meet the treatment guidelines, these should be documented as well.

Some facilities have experienced stroke teams available on a 24-hour basis that can perform urgent angiography on ischemic stroke patients. In these centers, intra-arterial tPA or angioplasty/ stenting of the specifically occluded vessel causing the stroke is possible.

If the emergency department concerned does not have adequate coverage by physicians experienced in stroke care and modern technology, there are several options:

- Choose not to accept patients suspected of having stroke and divert them to a nearby stroke center if one is available.
- Upgrade the facility to meet the standards and then accept patients. This requires improving technology, adding experienced stroke clinicians, and facilitating throughput.
- If it is not feasible to divert to a nearby facility, consider connecting with such a facility by telemedicine or consultative arrangements to facilitate care.

Whether or not tPA is given for the acute infarction, the patient should be admitted to the hospital to further investigate the etiology of the infarction (e.g. a cardiac embolic source, atrial fibrillation, vertebral-basilar atherosclerotic disease, etc.) and to aggressively treat ischemic risk factor.

Dr. Lee. Like Dr. Brazis, the stroke treatment protocols for reperfusion in acute ischemic stroke (including those producing a homonymous hemianopsia) are at the discretion of the stroke team. Typically the ophthalmologist is making the diagnosis, ordering the imaging study urgently, and then referring the patient to the stroke service. The primary acute imaging of choice remains the non-contrast head CT scan to exclude acute hemorrhage or a large volume infarction. Although cranial CT is superior to MRI for acute bleed, a CT scan is not as sensitive as MRI with specialized sequences (e.g. diffusion or perfusion imaging) for acute cerebral ischemia. Unfortunately, reperfusion therapy may be inadvertently given to patients with a "stroke mimic" (e.g. migraine or seizure related Todd's paralysis) and this decision is best left to the experts. Special MRI sequences based upon the restriction of the diffusion of water called diffusion-weighted imaging (DWI) can detect hyperacute ischemic stroke before structural change on CT or traditional MRI. In many of my patients who present with an acute, subacute or unknown duration for a homonymous hemianopsia, the CT scan is negative. If the initial CT is negative, then I typically recommend a cranial MRI with DWI sequences and contrast. If there is evidence for a prior old infarct but no acute infarct (negative DWI), then typically I will contact the stroke service by phone and let them proceed with an outpatient stroke evaluation at their individual discretion and timing rather than admit the patient.

2B

Acute Painful Homonymous Hemianopsia

CASE NO. 2B

A 37-year-old female was reaching up on a high shelf for a pack of cigarettes while at her job at a convenience store when she noted the acute onset of severe neck pain. Shortly after the pain developed, she noticed difficulty in seeing. She denied any periocular pain or headaches, weakness or photophobia. She could not recall any recent prior trauma. She went home "to sleep it off" but upon awakening the next day, she felt worse; she did not think that her vision was clear to the left side in both eyes.

Ocular examination showed a visual acuity of 20/20 in each eye. There was no relative afferent pupillary defect, ptosis or anisocoria. Ocular motility was full. Fundus examination was normal. Goldmann perimetry showed an almost complete, congruous, denser superiorly left homonymous hemianopia (Fig. 2B.1).

Dr. Lee. The localization of a homonymous hemianopia is a retrochiasmal lesion on the contralateral side. The absence of other neurologic symptoms suggests occipital rather than temporal or parietal lobe localization. The Goldmann visual field demonstrates an almost complete, congruous homonymous hemianopia without macular sparing or temporal crescent sparing. The acute onset suggests a vascular event (stroke or hemorrhage) rather than a neoplastic process or other etiology. In a young patient with neck pain, the major concerns would be vertebral arterial dissection with a

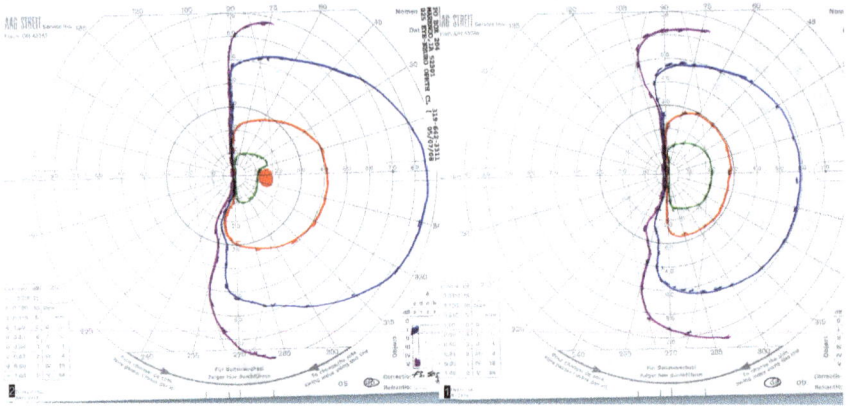

Fig. 2B.1. Goldmann perimetry showed a left almost complete homonymous hemianopia.

posterior cerebral artery infarct or thromboembolic disease. The first study should be cranial imaging. Typically in the emergency room a non-contrast CT scan of the head would be the first line imaging study followed by an MRI if the CT was negative. Diffusion weighted imaging (DWI) that demonstrates restricted diffusion of water (bright signal on DWI with matched dark signal on apparent diffusion coefficient or ADC map) in an acute stroke might be useful. Concomitant MRA of the head and neck might be useful to evaluate vascular abnormalities at the same time as the MRI. Admission to the hospital would be recommended if the patient had imaging evidence for an acute stroke.

Dr. Brazis. The patient needs urgent neuroimaging. However, if the deficit is due to an acute ischemic infarction, the patient does not satisfy the criteria for the injection of tissue plasminogen activator (tPA) because she is already beyond the therapeutic window for the use of this agent.

Course. Cranial MRI/MRA (Fig. 2B.2) showed a subacute infarction of the right PCA territory on DWI. Subsequent catheter angiography

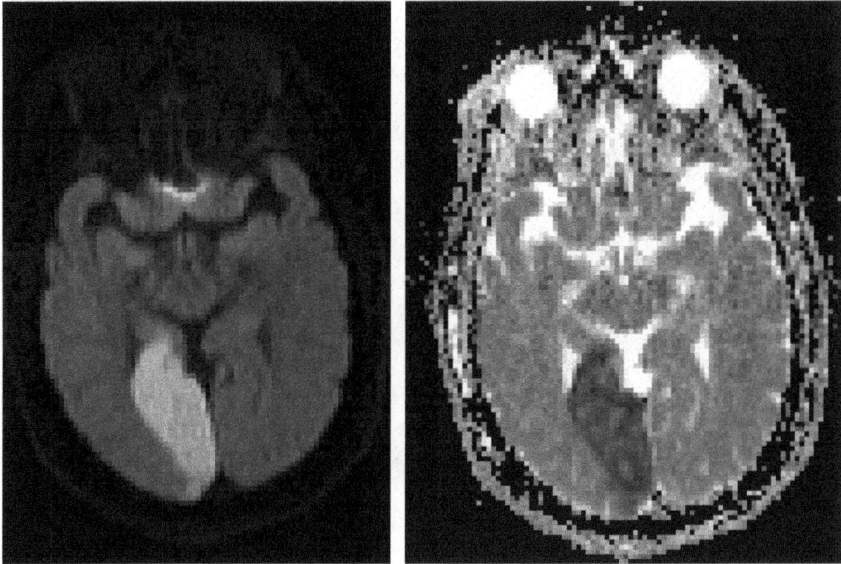

Fig. 2B.2. Diffusion weighted imaging (DWI) on MRI shows restricted diffusion (bright signal on right with dark signal on matched apparent diffusion coefficient (ADC) map consistent with a right posterior cerebral artery (PCA) distribution infarct.

showed a subtotal occlusion of the right vertebral consistent with a dissection. The patient was admitted to the stroke service and did well on antiplatelet therapy. The visual field loss, however, did not recover.

REFERENCES

Caplan LR. (2004) Thrombolysis 2004: The good, the bad and the ugly. *Rev Neurolog Dis* **1**:16–26.

Pessin MS, Lathi ES, Cohen MB, *et al*. (1987) Clinical features and mechanism of occipital infarction. *Ann Neurol* **21**:290–299.

National Institute of Neurologic Disorders and Stroke rt-PA Stroke Study Group. (1995) Tissue plasminogen activator for acute ischemic stroke. *N Engl J Med* **333**:1581–1587.

3A

Acute Bilateral Optic Disc Edema

CASE NO. 3A

A 31-year-old white female presented in the ER complaining of bilateral blurry vision for the previous two days. She also related mild headaches for the previous week. Past medical history was unremarkable. Her only medication was birth control pills. Family history was noncontributory.

On examination, the patient's visual acuity was 20/60 OD and 20/80 OS. Confrontation visual fields were normal in both eyes. The pupillary examination was normal without a relative afferent pupillary defect. Ocular motility was full. Slit lamp examination was unremarkable. Intraocular pressure was 12 mm Hg in each eye. Ophthalmoscopy showed bilateral optic nerve edema (Fig. 3A.1). The macula, vessels, and periphery were within normal limits.

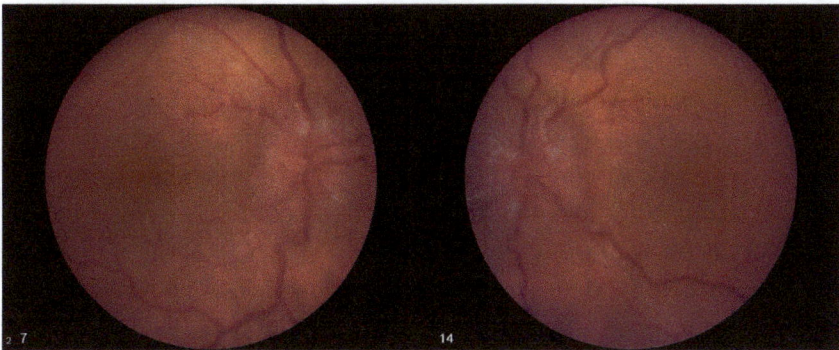

Fig. 3A.1. Fundus photography showing grade IV optic nerve edema bilaterally.

Discussion

Dr. Brazis. All patients with papilledema require a thorough urgent neurologic and neuro-ophthalmologic history and physical examination. In general, the syndromes causing increased intracranial pressure include:

- Primary causes
  - o Idiopathic pseudotumor cerebri syndrome (idiopathic intracranial hypertension) with or without papilledema

- Secondary causes
  - o Hydrocephalus
  - o Shunt failure in patient with hydrocephalus (ventriculomegaly may be absent)
  - o Mass lesions — tumor, hemorrhage, large infarction, abscess
  - o Meningitis/encephalitis
  - o Subarachnoid hemorrhage
  - o Trauma
  - o Arteriovenous malformations (AVM) with high blood flow overloading venous return
  - o Intracranial (e.g. cerebral venous sinuses) or extracranial (e.g. internal jugular) venous obstruction
  - o Secondary pseudotumor cerebri syndrome due to certain systemic diseases or drugs

In all patients with bilateral optic disc swelling, the blood pressure should be checked to evaluate for possible malignant hypertension. Blood dyscrasia should be considered if there are other suggestive retinal vascular findings (e.g. incomplete or complete central retinal vein occlusion with optic disc edema).

Neuroimaging is required in all patients. Cranial CT imaging is the preferred study in evaluating acute vascular processes (e.g. subarachnoid, epidural, subdural, or intracerebral hemorrhage, acute infarction) or in acute head trauma (e.g. rule out fracture, acute bleed). CT scan may be used in patients with contraindications to MR imaging (e.g. pacemakers, metallic clips in head, metallic foreign bodies), and markedly obese or claustrophobic patients who cannot have an MRI. Otherwise, MR imaging is the modality of choice in papilledema. MR angiography or MR venography may be useful for suspected arterial disease or venous obstruction. If neuroimaging shows no structural lesion or hydrocephalus, then lumbar puncture is warranted. Studies should include an accurate opening pressure, CSF cell count and differential, glucose, and protein. Additional CSF studies including cytology, syphilis testing, and other appropriate studies for microbial agents may also be performed.

Patients with a history of a ventriculoperitoneal shunt for hydrocephalus may develop papilledema, visual loss, or signs of a dorsal midbrain syndrome due to shunt failure. Usually CT or MR imaging reveals recurrence of the hydrocephalus. Shunt malfunction may occur without ventriculomegaly, perhaps due to poor ventricular compliance and "stiff ventricles." Shunt failure should thus be considered when there are signs or symptoms of increased intracranial pressure in a shunted patient even if ventriculomegaly is absent in order to prevent deterioration of visual function and potentially irreversible visual loss.

Pseudotumor cerebri (PTC), also known as idiopathic intracranial hypertension (IIH), is a diagnosis of exclusion, and the modified Dandy criteria include:

- Normal neuroimaging studies (usually MRI and MRV)
- Normal cerebrospinal fluid contents
- Elevated opening pressure
- Signs and symptoms related only to increased intracranial pressure (e.g. headache, papilledema, nonlocalizing sixth nerve palsy).

Pseudotumor cerebri (PTC) is usually idiopathic but may be secondary due to certain systemic diseases, drugs, pregnancy, and intracranial or extracranial venous obstruction. Obstruction or impairment of intracranial venous drainage may result in cerebral edema with increased intracranial pressure and papilledema. Tumors that occlude the posterior portion of the superior sagittal sinus or other cerebral venous sinuses may also cause increased intracranial pressure. Septic or aseptic thrombosis or ligation of the cavernous sinus, lateral sinus, sigmoid sinus, or superior sagittal sinus may mimic PTC. Ligation of one or both jugular veins (e.g. radical neck dissection), thrombosis of a central intravenous catheters in the chest or neck, compression of the jugular vein, hemodynamically significant left-to-right cardiac shunt from a cardiac septal defect, subclavian vein catheterization and arteriovenous fistula, the superior vena cava syndrome, or a glomus jugulare tumor impairing venous drainage may also cause increased ICP. Osteopetrosis causing obstruction of venous outflow at the jugular foramen has also been reported and depressed skull fracture with compression of the venous sinuses are other rare causes of increased ICP.

Cerebral venous sinus thrombosis (CVST) may be the mechanism for PTC reported in several conditions including: systemic lupus erythematosus, essential thrombocythemia, protein S deficiency, antithrombin III deficiency, the antiphospholipid antibody syndrome, activated protein C resistance, paroxysmal nocturnal hemoglobinuria, Behçet disease, meningeal sarcoidosis, lymphoma, hypervitaminosis A, mastoiditis, Lyme disease, and trichinosis.

CVST can present with all the classic criteria for idiopathic pseudotumor cerebri, including normal CT imaging and cerebrospinal fluid contents. In one study, of 160 consecutive patients with CVT, 59 patients (37%) presented with isolated intracranial hypertension. Neuroimaging revealed involvement of more than one venous sinus in 35 patients (59%); CT imaging was normal in 27 of 50 patients (54%). The superior sagittal sinus was involved in 32 patients (54%) (isolated in seven) and the lateral sinus in 47 (80%) (isolated in 17). The straight sinus was thrombosed in eight patients, cortical veins were involved in two, and deep cerebral veins in three, always in association with thrombosis in the superior sagittal sinus or lateral sinuses. Etiologic risk factors included local causes (7), surgery (1), inflammatory disease (18), infection (2), cancer (1), postpartum (1), coagulopathies (11), and oral contraception (7). The cause was unknown in 11 cases (19%). The authors emphasized that MR imaging and MR venography should be considered in presumed isolated intracranial hypertension.

Increased blood flow and venous hypertension have also been implicated as the mechanism of papilledema noted in some patients with cerebral arteriovenous malformations (AVMs), especially dural AVMs and fistulas. PTC may also occur in association with the Chiari I malformation.

Many systemic diseases, drugs, vitamin deficiencies and excesses, pregnancy, and hereditary conditions have been associated with secondary pseudotumor cerebri. In general, many of these reported associations may be coincidental and anecdotal. The etiologies most firmly associated include:

- **Drugs:** Hypervitaminosis A, steroid withdrawal, anabolic steroids, lithium, nalidixic acid, the insecticide chlordecone (Kepone), isoretinoin, ketaprofen (Orudis) or indomethacin in Bartter's syndrome, thyroid replacement in hypothyroid children, danazol, all-trans-retinoic acid (ATRA) or isotretinoin or tretinoin, cyclosporine, exogenous growth hormone, tetracycline, and minocycline.
- **Systemic diseases:** Behçet's syndrome, renal failure, Addison's disease, hypoparathyroidism, systemic lupus erythematosus, sarcoidosis.

In this patient, MRV revealed occlusion of the superior sagittal sinus (Figs. 3A.2 to 3A.4), perhaps induced by her birth control pills. A thrombotic profile to investigate for the presence of a prothrombotic state and a pregnancy test are indicated.

Some cases of PTC secondary to venous sinus obstruction may be successfully treated using angioplasty with venous sinus stenting or thrombolytic infusion to improve the venous outlet obstruction. Some authorities suggest anticoagulation. In all cases, if the papilledema persists, other treatments to protect vision should

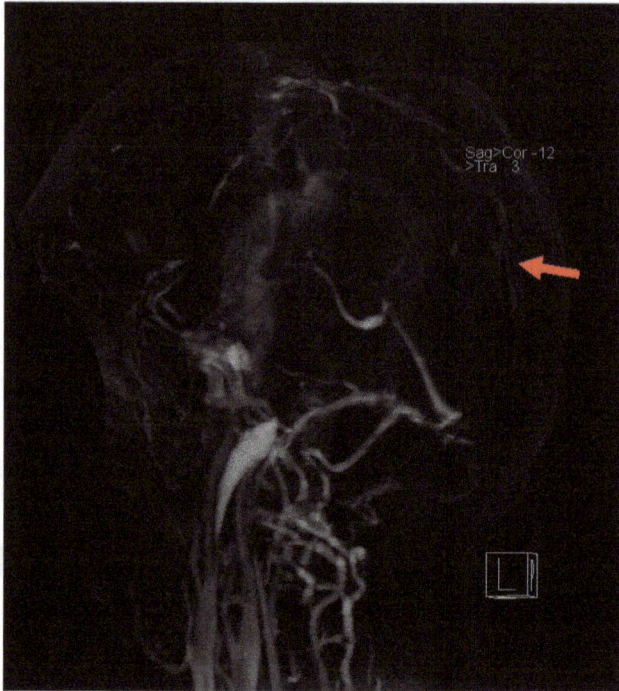

Fig. 3A.2. MR venogram pos contrast demonstrates occlusion of the superior sagittal sinus (*arrow*).

be considered, including surgical procedures such as optic nerve sheath fenestration, ventriculo-peritoneal shunt, or lumboperitoneal shunt.

Dr. Lee. My typical approach to a patient with papilledema is to look for an exogenous cause (e.g. medication induced PTC as described by Dr. Brazis above), assess for risk factors for cerebral venous sinus thrombosis (e.g. clotting disorders, trauma) and check the systemic blood pressure. In patients who fit the "demographic profile" for PTC (e.g. obese young female with signs and symptoms confined to those related to increased intracranial pressure), I then proceed with a cranial MRI and contrast MRV to rule out CVST. If

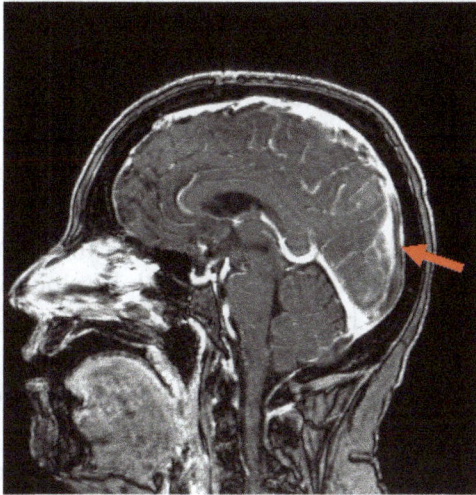

Fig. 3A.3. Brain MRI sagital T1 pos contrast demonstrates the absence of contrast in the superior sagittal sinus (*arrow*) consistent with the blood clot.

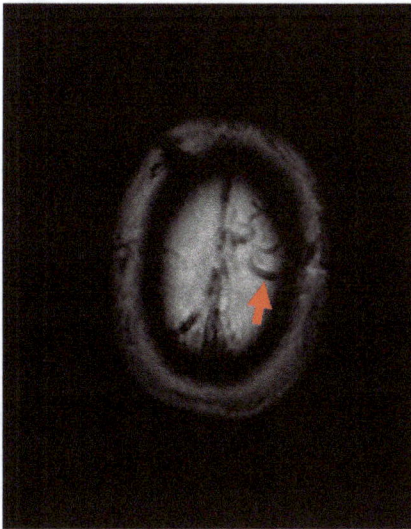

Fig. 3A.4. Brain MRI axial gradient demonstrates decreased signal within the cortical vein (*arrow*) consistent with the clot.

31

the MRI and MRV are negative, then I proceed to a lumbar puncture to check the cerebrospinal fluid (CSF) contents and to measure the opening pressure. I almost always initially treat patients with papilledema due to PTC with acetazolamide (Diamox) unless there is a contraindication. I perform a typical complete eye exam, a formal visual field, and document their baseline with fundus photography. Some obese female patients come to me with a previously performed normal contrast MRI but no MRV. In these patients, assuming they have no other atypical signs or symptoms, I will obtain the LP to confirm the diagnosis and treat as PTC. If they fail to respond appropriately or if they are not the typical PTC demographic (e.g. male, thin, elderly), I will ask the patient to undergo a contrast MRV to rule out sinus thrombosis. Unlike a typical idiopathic PTC patient who can be treated as outpatients generally, CVST patients usually require hospitalization and I contact my stroke neurology colleagues in this regard for decision making on admission and in patient medical treatment.

3B

Subacute Bilateral Optic Disc Edema

CASE NO. 3B

A 24-year-old woman presented with a six-week history of bifrontal headaches, pulse-synchronous tinnitus, and transient visual obscurations (TVOs) lasting seconds at a time OU. She rated her headache as severe (10/10 scale) and she was taking regular acetaminophen and ibuprofen for pain control without relief. The headaches were worse in the morning and when leaning forward. The TVOs were worse with bending over and seemed to be occurring more frequently. She has been feeling nauseated over the past two weeks but there were no additional neurological symptoms. Her vision has been getting blurred over the last 10 days and has deteriorated over the past 48 hours. She admits to a 52 lb weight gain over the past three months which had occurred after the birth of her last child. Her current height was 5'5" and she weighed 312 lb.

There was no significant past medical history and there was no positive family history of headaches. She was not allergic to any medication and other than oral analgesics, she was not on any regular medication. She specifically denied the use of tetracyclines, lithium, vitamin A analogs, or corticosteroids (typically withdrawal from steroid treatment).

Examination revealed a moderately obese young woman. The blood pressure was 130/85 mm Hg. Visual acuity was 20/200 OU. She had no diplopia and there was no evidence for sixth nerve palsy on exam. Fundus examination (Figs. 3B.1 and 3B.2) showed severe optic nerve head edema with hemorrhages and OCT confirmed

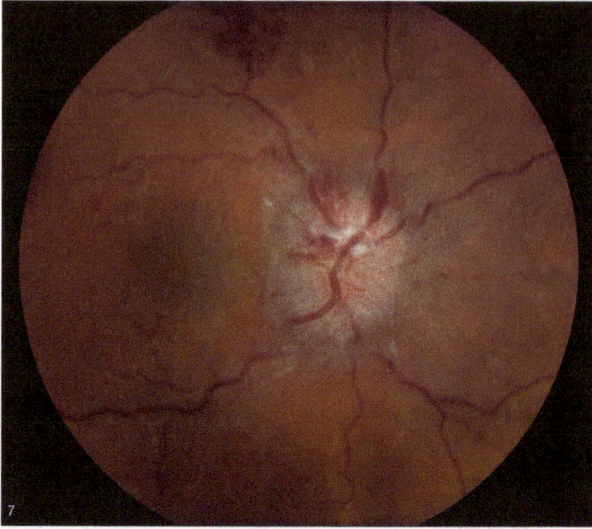

Fig. 3B.1. Color picture of the right fundus showing optic disc swelling with overlying hemorrhages.

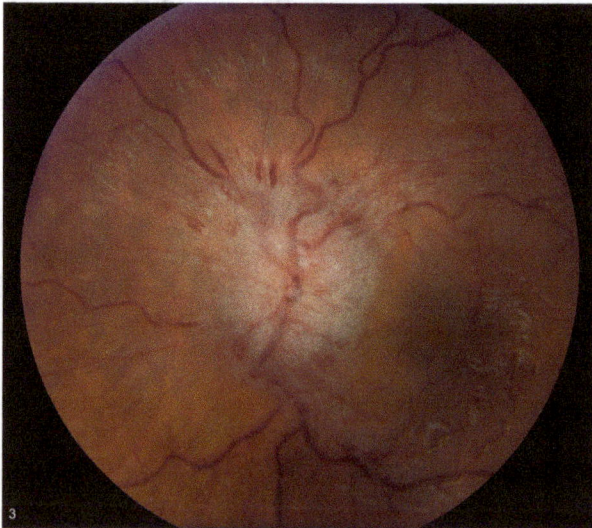

Fig. 3B.2. Color picture of the left fundus showing optic disc swelling with overlying hemorrhages.

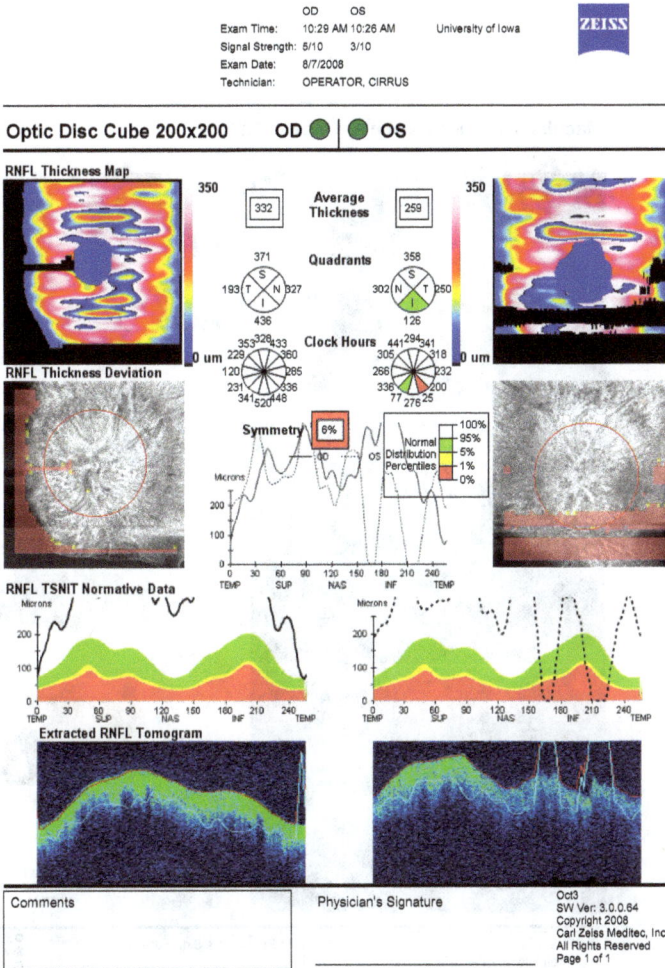

Fig. 3B.3. Optic nerve head OCT showing gross bilateral swelling of the optic nerve heads.

serous fluid in the macula OU (Figs. 3B.3–3B.5). Goldmann perimetry showed the presence of central scotoma and enlarged blind spots OU (Figs. 3B.6 and 3B.7). The remainder of the eye and neurologic exam was normal.

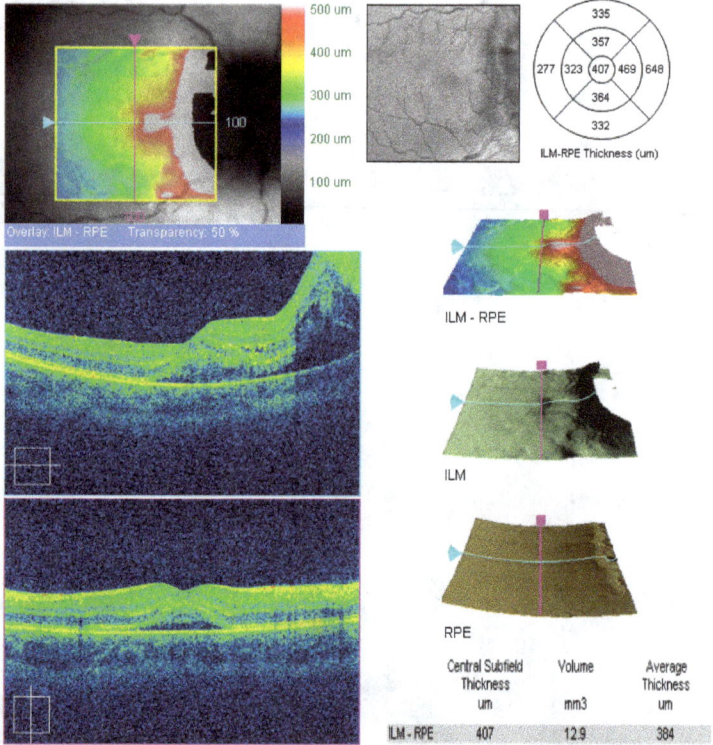

Fig. 3B.4. Macular OCT of the right eye showing serous fluid extending to the macula.

Discussion

Dr. Lee. Bilateral optic disc edema in the setting of headache, TVOs, and pulse synchronous tinnitus (PST) should be considered to be

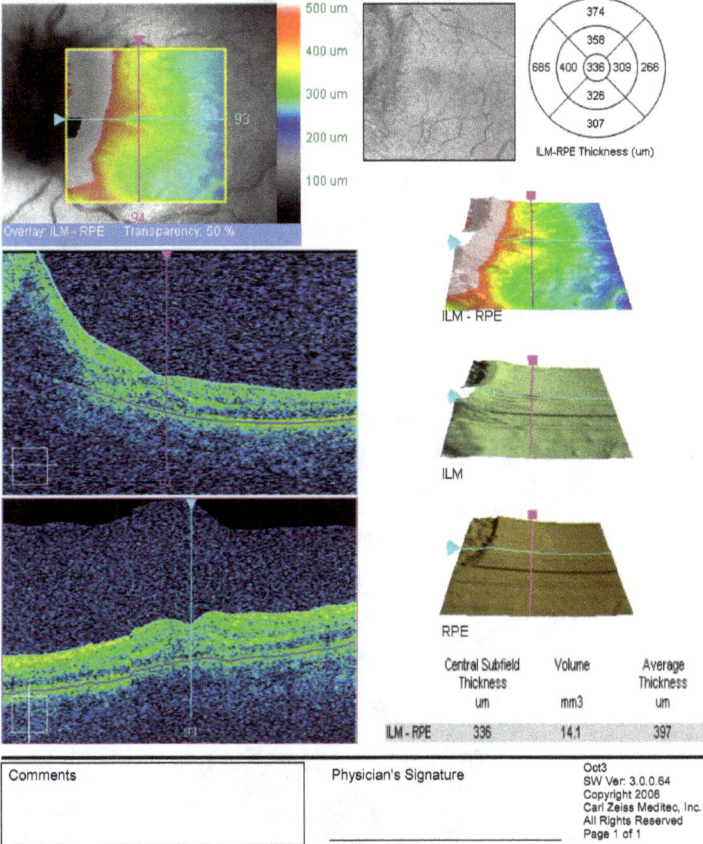

Fig. 3B.5. Macular OCT of the left eye showing serous fluid extending to the macula.

papilledema until proven otherwise. The clinician is encouraged to limit the use of the term "papilledema" for optic disc edema related to increased intracranial pressure (ICP). This will avoid miscommunication with other physicians. In an obese female, the

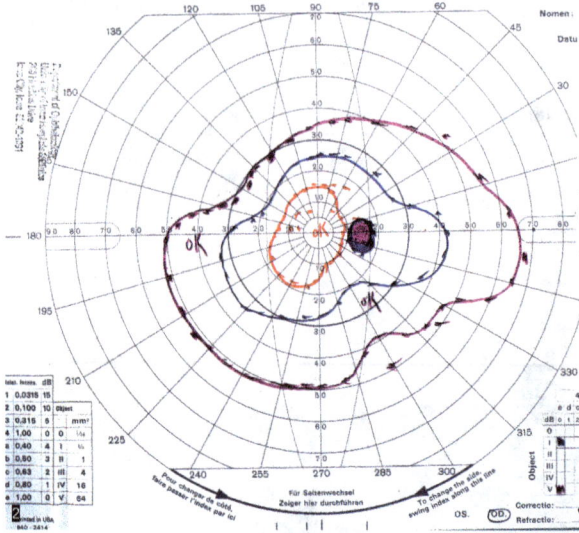

Fig. 3B.6. Goldmann perimetry of the right eye showing enlargement of the blind spot and constriction of the field.

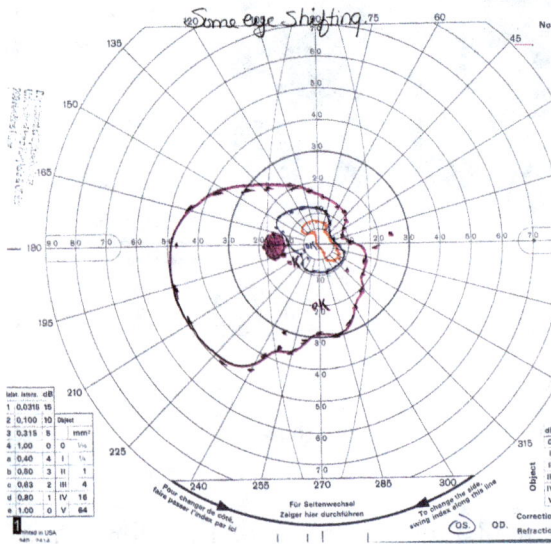

Fig. 3B.7. Goldmann perimetry of the left eye showing a central scotoma and constriction of the field.

diagnosis of idiopathic PTC should be cosnsidered as the leading diagnosis.

As noted above I recommend neuroimaging (e.g. contrast MRI with MRV) and a LP to confirm the diagnosis of idiopathic PTC. I recommend medical therapy with acetazolamide (Diamox) as our first line treatment. Other diuretics and other medical treatments can be used as adjunctive treatments (e.g. furosemide, topirimate) but acetazolamide is my preferred first line agent. If patients fail, are intolerant to, or non-compliant with maximum medical therapy, then consideration could be given for surgical treatment (i.e. optic nerve sheath fenestration [ONSF] or intracranial shunting procedure). I tend to favor ONSF for patients with visual loss as their predominant complaint and shunting procedure for those with headache or headache with severe visual loss as their predominant complaint. The choice between lumboperitoneal shunt (LPS) and stereotactic ventriculoperitoneal shunt (VPS) with or without a programmable valve must be made on an individual and institutional basis, depending on local availability and expertise with each procedure. In patients such as this case who present with visual loss, the etiology for the visual loss should be carefully established. Patients with severe visual field loss or central acuity loss (not attributable to macular fluid or hemorrhage) should be considered for emergent surgical intervention (e.g. ONSF, LPS, or VPS). The most common errors made in patients with IIH include not excluding alternative etiologies especially in patients who do not fit the typical IIH profile (e.g. thin patients, males, elderly or children); and ordering the wrong or inadequate neuroimaging study (I recommend contrast cranial MRI and MRV unless there is a contraindication). A CT with CT venogram is sometimes a necessary alternative imaging choice for patients who cannot have an MRI (e.g. pacemaker, severe claustrophobia, metallic foreign body, etc.).

Dr. Brazis. I agree with Dr. Lee that idiopathic PTC is a diagnosis of exclusion. The modified Dandy criteria include: 1) normal neuroimaging studies (usually MRI); 2) normal cerebrospinal fluid contents; 3) elevated opening pressure; and 4) signs and symptoms related only to increased intracranial pressure (e.g. headache, papilledema, nonlocalizing sixth nerve palsy). Pseudotumor cerebri (PTC) is usually idiopathic but may be due to certain systemic diseases, drugs, pregnancy, and intracranial or extracranial venous obstruction.

I recommend that patients with PTC undergo MR imaging of the head. Atypical patients should undergo MR venography to evaluate for venous occlusive disease but we recommend cerebral angiography only in select cases. If venous occlusive disease is discovered, then evaluation for a hypercoaguable state and vasculitis should be performed.

My indications for surgical treatment (usually optic nerve sheath fenestration or ventriculoperitoneal shunt) for PTC include:

- New worsening visual field defect[a]
- Enlargement of previously existing visual field defect[a]
- Reduced visual acuity not due to macular edema
- Presence of severe visual loss (20/40 or worse) in one or both eyes at time of initial examination
- Anticipated hypotension induced by treatment of high blood pressure or renal dialysis
- Psychosocial reasons, such as patient's inability to perform visual field studies, noncompliance with medications, an itinerant lifestyle
- Headache unresponsive to standard headache medications

Course. A cranial MRI with contrast MRV demonstrated an empty sella and the edematous nerve heads were also visible (Figs. 3B.8 and 3B.9). There was no evidence for cranial venous sinus thrombosis. A lumbar puncture showed an opening pressure of 30 cm of water but normal cerebrospinal fluid (CSF) contents. The patient was

---

[a]Blind spot enlargement should not be considered significant visual loss (refractive).

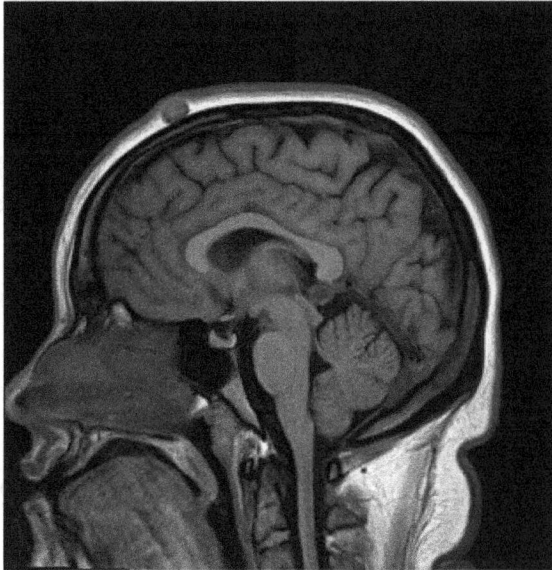

Fig. 3B.8. Sagittal MRI showing an empty sella.

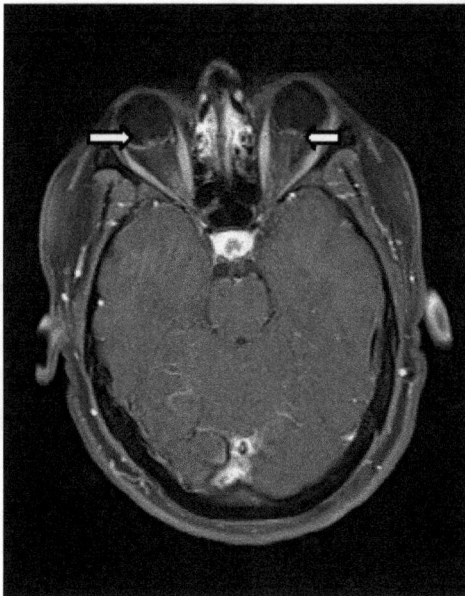

Fig. 3B.9. Axial MRI showing edematous optic discs in both eyes labeled with arrows.

started on acetazolamide 500 mg TID but the disc edema persisted and she underwent optic nerve sheath fenestration OD. After surgery the disc edema improved dramatically, the headache resolved, and the vision returned to 20/40 OU with a mild residual relative central scotoma OU. The serous macular fluid resolved but she was left with moderate retinal pigment epithelium (RPE) changes OU in the macula.

REFERENCES

Biousse V, Ameri A, Bousser M-G. (1999) Isolated intracranial hypertension as the only sign of cerebral venous thrombosis. *Neurology* **53**:1537–1542.

Lin A, Foroozan R, Danesh-Meyer HV, *et al.* (2006) Occurrence of cerebral venous sinus thrombosis in patients with presumed idiopathic intracranial hypertension. *Ophthalmology* **113**:2281–2284.

Sylaja PN, Ahsan Moosa NV, Radhakrishnan K, *et al.* (2003) Differential diagnosis of patients with intracranial sinus venous thrombosis related isolated intracranial hypertension from those with idiopathic intracranial hypertension. *J Neurol Sci* **215**:9–12.

4

Acute Homonymous Hemianopsia in Febrile Patient

CASE NO. 4

A 22-year-old white female presented in the ER complaining of high fever and chills after undergoing a piercing in her nose (Fig. 4.1). She also related some difficulty with her vision on her left side. Past medical history was unremarkable. On examination her visual acuity was 20/20 in each eye. Ocular motility was full in both eyes. Pupillary examination was normal. The Goldmann visual field showed an inferior left homonymous hemianopia (Fig. 4.2). Slit lamp examination was unremarkable. Ophthalmoscopy was within normal limits.

Discussion

Dr. Brazis. An inferior homonymous quadrantanopia is most often due to a superior occipital lesion or a parietal lesion. In patients with occipital lesions, the field defects often occur in isolation, while other localizing signs or parietal involvement are usually evident in patients with parietal lesions. Therefore, although visual field defects may occur in relative isolation with parietal lobe lesions, lesions in this location more often betray themselves by other signs of neurologic dysfunction. Parietal lobe lesions may be associated with contralateral somatosensory impairment, including impaired object recognition, impaired position sense, impaired touch and pain sensation, and tactile extinction. Dominant parietal

43

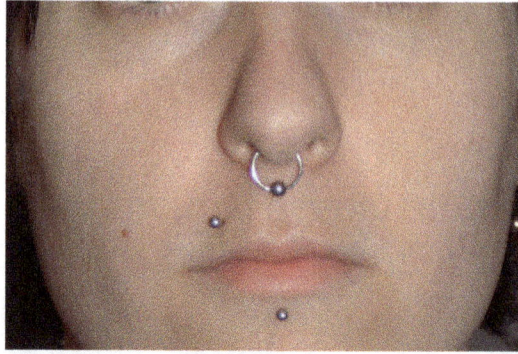

Fig. 4.1. External photography showing the nose piercing.

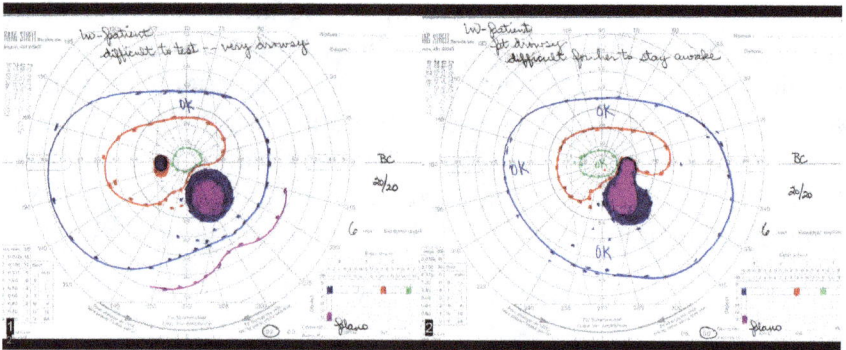

Fig. 4.2. Goldman visual field showing the inferior right homonymous hemianopia.

lesions may cause apraxia, finger agnosia, acalculia, right-left disorientation, alexia, and aphasic disturbances. Non-dominant lesions may be associated with a anosognosia (denial of neurologic impairment), autotopagnosia (failure to recognize himiplegic limbs as belonging to the self), spatial disorientation, hemispatial neglect, constructional apraxia (abnormal drawing and copying), and dressing apaxia.

In a patient with fever and chills and a visual field defect, one must be concerned about the possibility of an infectious process affecting the central nervous system. Lesions producing such impairment include abscesses, aneurysms, empyema, encephalitis, granuloma, meningitis, and ischemic infarction related to endocarditis or sepsis.

An abscess is a circumscribed area of pus that may be epidural, subdural, or intracerebral. Intracerebral abscesses are usually solitary and are most often located in the cerebral hemispheres. Most intracranial abscesses are caused either by local invasion of one or more organisms or by septic emboli. An untreated or incompletely treated middle ear infection is the most common source of a locally derived brain abscess. Chronic mastoiditis may produce brain abscess as may chronic paranasal sinusitis. Orbital cellulitis may cause intracranial abscess but these are usually frontal or temporal in location caused by extension of the organism through the superior orbital fissure. Acute bacterial meningitis is a rare cause of brain abscess except in neonates. Septic foci on the scalp or face are relatively rare cause of brain abscess. Dental infections, tonsillitis, or other facial infections may cause an abscess. Cerebral abscesses may also occur after trauma or neurosurgical procedures. Metastatic abscess seas that result from blood-borne organisms may develop in the setting of bacteremia or septicemia. Such abscesses are usually multiple and may be of varying size.

Most intracranial abscesses are caused by bacteria. Aerobic bacteria are found more often than anaerobic bacteria, but polymicrobial infections may exist in a single abscess. The most common aerobic bacteria that produce both single and multiple intracranial abscess are Gram-positive cocci, such as *Streptococcus* and *Staphlococcus* species, and Gram-negative bacilli, including *Haemophilus* species and many members of the Enterobacteriaceae. Nevertheless, Gram-negative cocci, such as *Neisseria meningitides*, and Gram-positive bacilli, such as *Listeria monocytogenes*, Actinomycosis, and *Nocardia*, can produce brain abscess in otherwise healthy people. The most common anaerobic bacteria that cause brain abscesses are the Gram-negative bacilli, *Bacteroides* and *Propionibacterium*. Organisms other than bacteria may produce intracranial abscesses, particularly in chronically ill, immunodeficient, or immunosuppressive patients. These include fungi, toxoplasmosis, *Cysticercus* species, *Angiostrongylus cantonensis,* and *Treponema pallidum.*

Neuroimaging, preferably contrast MRI studies, are warranted urgently. Suppurative encephalitis appears as an area of decreased density on a CT scan, whereas an abscess appears as a low-density core surrounded by a capsule that enhances when the patient is given an intravenous injection of iodinated contrast agent. Features of abscess on MRI study include:

- Peripheral edema producing mild hypointensity on T1-weighted images and marked hyperintensity on proton density-weighted and T2-weighted images;
- Central necrosis with abscess fluid that is hypointense relative to white matter and hyperintense relative to CSF on T1-weighted images and hyperintense relative to gray matter on proton density-weighted and T2-weighted images;
- Extraparenchymal spread (intraventricular or subarachnoid) manifested by increased intensity relative to normal CSF on T1-weighted images, proton density-weighted, and T2 weighted images;
- Visualization of the abscess capsule is iso- or mildly hyperintense relative to brain on T1-weighted image and iso- to hypointense related to white matter on proton density-weighted and T2-weighted images.

Course. Initial acute brain CT with contrast in our patient demonstrated a ring enhancing lesion in the left occiptal lobe consistent with brain abscess (Fig. 4.3). Diffusion-weighted image (DWI) MRI of the brain demonstrates high signal in the left occipital region corresponding to the area of ring enhancement, representing pus within the abscess (Fig. 4.4). It is thought that the abscess was due to infection from the patient's recent nose piercing.

Dr. Brazis. The treatment of an intracranial abscess is directed both at the abscess and its source, and may be medical, surgical, or both.

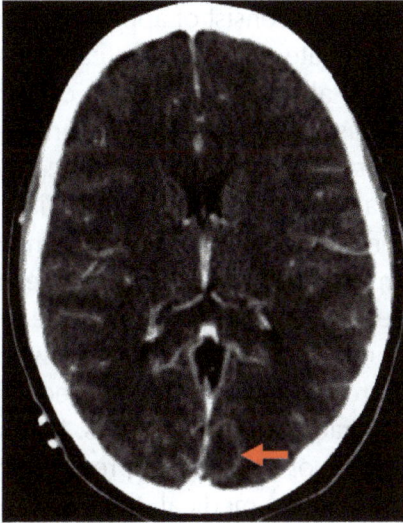

Fig. 4.3. Brain CT with contrast demonstrates the ring lesion in the left occiptal lobe (*arrow*) consistent with brain abscess.

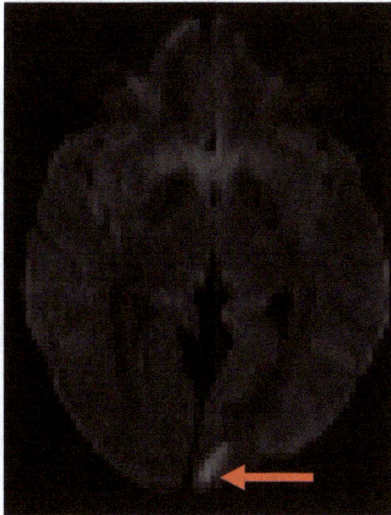

Fig. 4.4. Diffusion-weighted image of the brain demonstrates high signal in the left occipital region (*arrow*) corresponding to the area of ring enhancement on the previous image representing an abscess.

Medical treatments usually consist of appropriate antibiotics or other drugs designed to eliminate the organism causing the infection. The blood brain barrier is altered in areas of cerebritis and abscess, thus allowing increased penetration of anti-infectious agents. Occasionally, corticosteroids are used to reduce the cerebral edema surrounding the intracranial abscess. The specific medical regimen recommended depends on the known or presumed causative organism. In patients with no significant neurologic deficits with a normal state of consciousness, with a single deep abscess less than 2 cm in diameter, harboring multiple abscesses, or for whom surgery of any type might be inappropriately hazardous, medical treatment alone may be successful in eradicating the abscess. If there is clinical deterioration, if CT scanning or MR imaging reveals enlargement of the abscess at any time during medical treatment, or if there is no decrease in size of the abscess within several weeks, surgery should be considered. Most patients with an intracerebral abscess should undergo aspiration or excision of the abscess for both diagnosis and treatment. Aspiration is usually all that is required. When a brain abscess results from a systemic infection, the source of infection also must be treated (e.g. bacterial endocarditis).

Dr. Lee. An intracerebral abscess can be a life-threatening condition. Although the classic triad of fever, headache and focal neurologic deficit (e.g. homonymous hemianopsia) are useful findings, these findings do not always occur in patients with a brain abscess. Likewise, an elevated white blood cell count or elevated erythrocyte sedimentation rate is only variably present if at all. Classically, a ring-enhancing mass lesion on CT or contrast MRI could be an abscess, a primary brain tumor or a metastasis. DWI in a brain abscess might show hyperintense signal as opposed to the other lesions in the differential, which normally would not be bright on DWI. A patient thought to have a primary brain tumor might undergo a biopsy alone and be discharged pending the pathology if an abscess is not considered ahead of time in the differential diagnosis. The absence of fever, headache, or leukocytosis provides a false sense of security in such patients. The history of piercing in this case is intriguing and brain abscess has been associated with tongue piercing.

REFERENCES

Haimes AB, Zimmerman RD, Morgello S, *et al.* (1989) MR imaging of brain abscesses. *AJR* **152**:1073–1085.

Irie H, Hasuo K, Yasumori K, *et al.* (1991) MRI of brain abscesses. *Nippon Acta Radiol* **51**:115–120.

Jacobson DM. (1997) The localizing value of quadrantanopia. *Arch Neurol* **54**:401–404.

5

Acute Painless Isolated Sixth Nerve Palsy

CASE NO. 5

A 66-year-old white man presented in the ER complaining of new onset binocular horizontal diplopia which was painless. He had no other eye complaints. His past medical history was remarkable for hypercholesterolemia controlled with statin therapy. Past medical, social, surgical, and family history were all non-contributory.

On examination, visual acuity was 20/20 in each eye. Confrontation visual field was normal in both eyes. Pupillary examination was normal without an afferent pupillary defect. Ocular motility showed isolated VI nerve palsy on the left (Fig. 5.1). There were 10–12 diopters of esotropia in primary position. Funduscopic

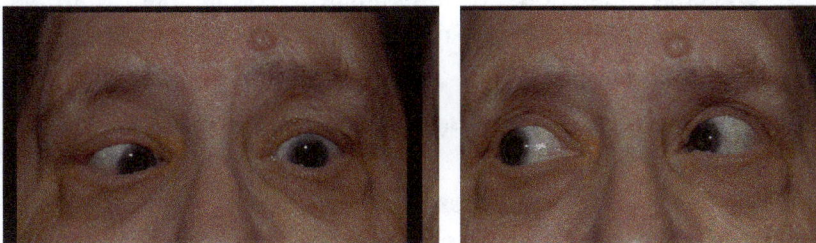

Fig. 5.1. Ocular motility photography showing the incomitant esotropia and the left abduction deficit in left gaze consistent with the left VI nerve palsy. Right gaze is normal.

examination showed a cup-to-disc ratio of 0.3 in each eye. The macula, vessels and periphery were normal in both eyes.

Discussion

Dr. Brazis. Based on topographic anatomy, sixth nerve palsies (SNPs) may be divided into isolated SNPs and non-isolated SNPs. The criteria for the diagnosis of an isolated SNP include:

- An ipsilateral abduction deficit
- Incomitant esodeviation that is typically worsened with gaze into the field of the weak lateral rectus muscle (may become comitant over time)
- Exclusion of Duane's retraction syndrome, spasm of the near reflex, and other causes of abduction deficits that can mimic a SNP, and exclusion of patients with signs of the following:
  1. Orbital disease (e.g. chemosis, proptosis, lid swelling, injection, and positive forced ductions)
  2. Myasthenia gravis (e.g. ptosis, Cogan's lid twitch sign, orbicularis oculi weakness, muscle fatigue or variability)
  3. Multiple cranial nerve palsies (including bilateral SNP) or radiculopathy
  4. Brainstem signs (e.g. Horner's syndrome, hemiplegia, cerebellar signs)
  5. Systemic, infectious, or inflammatory risk factors for an SNP (e.g. history of previous malignancy, giant cell arteritis, collagen vascular disease)
- Exclusion of patients with severe headache

There are a number of types of SNP that help to differentiate etiology and guide the management of SNP.

Type 1: Non-isolated SNP

- SNP are considered non-isolated in the presence of the exclusionary conditions outlined above.

Type 2: Traumatic SNP

- Isolated unilateral SNP, which have a clearly established temporal relationship to significant previous head trauma and do not progress, are considered traumatic in origin. Patients with SNP following minor head trauma are excluded.

Type 3: Congenital SNP

- Patients born with SNP or noted to have a SNP within the first three months of life.

Type 4: Vasculopathic SNP

- Vasculopathic SNP occur in patients older than 55 years or those with known ischemic risk factors (e.g. hypertension or diabetes).

Type 5: Nonvasculopathic SNP

- Patients without vasculopathic risk factors defined above are considered to have nonvasculopathic SNP.

Type 6: Progressive (non-isolated) or Unresolved SNP

- SNP that worsen after the acute stage (greater than two weeks) as defined by a significant increase in the measured ocular deviation or who develop new neurologic findings are considered progressive or non-isolated. Patients without resolution in the measured horizontal deviation after 12 to 16 weeks are considered unresolved.

The first clinical step is to determine whether the sixth nerve palsy is indeed occurring in isolation. Sixth nerve nuclear lesions involve the projections to the contralateral third nerve nucleus via the medial longitudinal fasciculus (MLF) and therefore cause a horizontal gaze palsy, rather than an isolated abduction deficit. An ipsilateral facial palsy may also occur because of the close proximity of the facial and abducens nerve in the pons. Nuclear lesions are usually associated with other brainstem signs (e.g. hemiparesis, hemisensory loss, a central Horner's syndrome). Likewise, lesions of the sixth nerve fascicle involve adjacent structures (e.g. cranial nerves V, VII, and VIII; cerebellar ataxia; a central Horner's syndrome; or contralateral hemiplegia). Patients with a presumed nuclear or fascicular SNP should undergo neuroimaging (usually magnetic resonance imaging) directed to the pons.

Lesions of the sixth nerve in the subarachnoid space may result in unilateral or bilateral SNP. This SNP can be a nonlocalizing finding due to increased intracranial pressure from any etiology. Patients with a subarachnoid space lesion should undergo neuroimaging directed to this location, followed by a lumbar puncture as needed.

Lesions of the petrous apex causing SNP are associated with other neurologic findings, including involvement of other cranial nerves (e.g. fifth, seventh, and eighth) or facial pain. Neuroimaging should be directed toward the petrous apex (MR imaging or computed tomography for bone involvement).

With lesions of the cavernous sinus, SNPs usually occur in association with other cranial neuropathies (e.g. third, fourth, or fifth nerves) or a Horner's syndrome. Neuroimaging (usually MR imaging) should be directed to the cavernous sinus.

Lesions of the orbit causing SNP are usually associated with other orbital signs such as proptosis or chemosis. Neuroimaging (preferably MR imaging) should be directed to the orbit.

Our patient had no history of a congenital SNP, had no history of recent trauma, and clinically has an isolated sixth nerve palsy. The patient may well have a vasculopathic (ischemic) SNP. Isolated vasculopathic SNP (Type 4) may be observed (without neuroimaging) for improvement for four to 12 weeks. Some authors have recommended observing vasculopathic isolated SNP beyond a three-month interval of recovery if the esotropia and the abduction deficit were decreasing. Elderly patients who present with an isolated SNP and headache, scalp tenderness, jaw claudication, or visual loss should undergo an appropriate evaluation for giant cell arteritis. We recommend erythrocyte sedimentation rate and, when clinically indicated, a temporal artery biopsy. Patients with progression or lack of improvement (Type 6) should undergo MRI neuroimaging.

It should be noted that early progression of paresis over one week in vasculopathic SNP is not uncommon. We do not consider progression over the first week after onset to be a sign of non-vasculopathic SNP.

I recommend that patients with nonvasculopathic SNP (Type 5) should undergo neuroimaging. Younger patients, or those without vasculopathic risk factors (Type 5), could also undergo a more extensive evaluation including a fasting blood glucose, complete blood cell count, and blood pressure check for underlying vasculopathy. Other testing including neuroimaging (MR imaging) and, if necessary, lumbar puncture are recommended. Type 5 SNPs have a significant (27%) chance of harboring an underlying malignant neoplasm. Evaluation for myasthenia gravis should also be considered in these patients. Testing for vasculopathic risk factors in Type 4 or Type 5 SNP patients should be performed, even in the absence of a previous history of diabetes or hypertension. Ocular motor cranial neuropathies may be the presenting or only sign of underlying vasculopathy in these patients.

Patients with progressive or unresolved SNPs (Type 6), or patients with new neurological signs or symptoms, should undergo neuroimaging. Progressive, or unresolved SNP patients, should have neuroimaging. In a study of 13 chronic SNPs, four were idiopathic, four were due to tumor, two were traumatic, one was postspinal anesthesia, one was due to temporal arteritis, and one was due to an intracavernous aneurysm. In this study, chronic was defined as an SNP lasting six months or longer. In another review of 38 patients with chronic SNP, 14 (37%) were discovered to have an intracranial lesion. These authors specifically recommended neuroradiologic investigation at onset in any patient with a history of carcinoma.

Aneurysm is a rare cause of acquired SNP. We do not typically recommend evaluation for aneurysm in isolated SNP but aneurysm can cause SNP in patients with signs of subarachnoid hemorrhage, papilledema, or other cranial neuropathies.

Dr. Lee. The traditional teaching is that an isolated SNP in a vasculopath that is resolving or has resolved does not need neuroimaging or other evaluation besides treatment of the vasculopathic risk factors. Some authors, given the low risk of MRI, disagree however with this "traditional" teaching. In several papers, a low but not zero rate of treatable etiologies (e.g. meningioma, brainstem ischemia, demyelinating disease) have been discovered through imaging at onset. Although I recognize the results of these studies, I personally still hold to the traditional approach as the most cost-effective means of evaluating isolated acute and presumed vasculopathic palsies. It has been my experience that vasculopathic patients with SNP who are also harboring an underlying nonischemic intracranial etiology either have non-neurologically isolated SNP or do not improve over the observational period and therefore will eventually undergo the appropriate imaging study. In these patients with meningiomas and other chronic lesions, the short delay in the diagnosis does not generally change management.

On the other hand, the chronic SNP is a well known "harbinger" of serious and potentially treatable intracranial disease. I image with cranial MRI with contrast and with constructive interference in steady state (CISS) sequences to follow the entire course of the sixth cranial nerve. Patients who worsen, do not improve, are not isolated, or who develop new neurologic signs and symptoms should undergo evaluation, including neuroimaging for alternative etiologies for the sixth nerve dysfunction.

REFERENCES

Galetta SL, Smith JL. (1989) Chronic isolated sixth nerve palsies. *Arch Neurol* **46**:79–82.

Jacobson DM. (1996) Progressive ophthalmoplegia with acute ischemic abducens nerve palsies. *Am J Ophthalmol* **122**:278–279.

Patel SV, Mutyala S, Leske DA, *et al.* (2004) Incidence, associations, and evaluation of sixth nerve palsy using a population-based method. *Ophthalmology* **111**:369–375.

Savino PJ, Hilliker JK, Casell GH, *et al.* (1982) Chronic sixth nerve palsies: Are they really harbingers of serious intracranial disease? *Arch Ophthalmol* **100**:1442–1444.

6

Acute Progressive Bilateral Ophthalmoplegia with Mental Status Change

CASE NO. 6

A 33-year-old man was brought to the ER because of a change in his mental status. His wife related that the patient was fine the previous day. However, on that day that he was brought in for evaluation, she noticed his confusion. His past medical history was remarkable for hypertension controlled with hydrochlorothiazide, and high cholesterol controlled with diet and exercise.

On examination, the patient was somnolent and also confused on attempts to measure his visual acuity. The ocular motility showed limitation of up-gaze. Pupillary examination showed light-near dissociation of the pupils OU. Slit lamp examination and funduscopic examinations were within normal limits.

Discussion

Dr. Brazis. The acute onset of mental status changes and ocular signs is most consistent with a cerebral infarct or hemorrhage. The impairment of upward gaze and the light-near dissociation of the pupils may be localized to the dorsal midbrain. With the dorsal midbrain syndrome, there is impairment of all upward eye movements (although the vestibuloocular reflex and Bell's phenomenon may sometimes be spared). Down-gaze saccades and smooth pursuit may be impaired, but downward vestibuloocular movements are spared.

Downbeating nystagmus may be present. The upper eyelid may be retracted, baring the sclera above the cornea (Collier's "tucked lid" sign); this sign is probably due to damage to posterior commissure levator inhibitory fibers or is a manifestation of normal levator — superior rectus synkinesis. Bilateral ptosis may result when the lesion extends ventrally to involve the caudal central nucleus of cranial nerve III. The pupils are large and react poorly to light, but the near response is spared (light-near dissociation). Occasionally, skew deviation with the higher eye on the side of the lesion is noted. Convergence and divergence are often impaired. In some patients, convergence spasm may result in slow or restricted abduction ("midbrain pseudo-sixth") during horizontal refixations. Attempted up-gaze may result in convergence-retraction nystagmus, with quick adducting-retraction jerks. This phenomenon can be elicited at the bedside by having the patient watch a downward-moving optokinetic drum. In this case, the normal upward corrective saccades are replaced by convergence-retractory nystagmus, which is made up not by convergence movements but by opposed adducting saccades at least in some cases. The retraction of the eye into the orbit results from irregular co-firing of several extraocular muscles perhaps due to impairment of recurrent inhibition with the oculomotor subnuclei or abnormal vergence activity. Fixation instability with square-wave jerks may also be noted.

Tumors are most often responsible for damage of the dorsal midbrain. Hydrocephalus is another common etiology, especially when dilation of the third ventricle and aqueduct or enlargement of the suprapineal recess causes pressure on and deformity of the posterior commissure. Patients with shunted hydrocephalus may develop features of the pretectal syndrome with shunt dysfunction even without any dilation of the ventricular system or elevation of intracranial pressure; thus, the observation of these clinical features provides a sensitive index of shunt dysfunction regardless of ventricular size or isolated measurements of intracranial pressure. Less common causes of pretectal syndrome include thalamic or midbrain hemorrhage or infarction, hypoxia, multiple sclerosis, trauma, lipid storage diseases, Wilson's disease, drugs (e.g. barbiturates, carbamazepine, neuroleptics), Whipple's disease, syphilis, and tuberculosis. Upward gaze is often limited in Parkinson's disease and may be rarely affected with vitamin B12 deficiency.

Occlusive vascular disease of the rostral basilar artery, usually embolic, frequently results in the "top of the basilar" syndrome due to infarction of the midbrain, thalamus, and portions of the temporal and occipital lobes. This syndrome may also occur in patients with giant basilar artery tip aneurysms, in patients with vasculitis, and after cerebral angiography. This syndrome variably includes:

- Disorders of eye movements: Unilateral or bilateral paralysis of upward or downward gaze, disordered convergence, pseudo-abducens palsy, convergence-retraction nystagmus, ocular abduction abnormalities, elevation and retraction of the upper eyelids (Collier's sign), skew deviation, and lightning-like eye oscillations.
- Pupillary abnormalities: Small and reactive, large or midposition and fixed, light-near dissociation, corectopia, occasionally oval pupil.
- Behavioral abnormalities: Somnolence, peduncular hallucinosis, memory difficulties, agitated delirium.
- Visual defects: Homonymous hemianopia, cortical blindness, Balint syndrome.
- Motor and sensory deficits.

Course. Indeed, the patient's MRI demonstrates restricted diffusion within the thalami bilaterally, consistent with acute ischemia (Fig. 6.1A). Circle of Willis 3D MIP angiography demonstrated complete occlusion of the distal basilar artery (Fig. 6.1B).

If the criteria for intravenous or intra-arterial tPA are satisfied (see Case No. 2) and the deficit was less than three hours in duration, tPA treatment should be considered. Whether tPA is given or

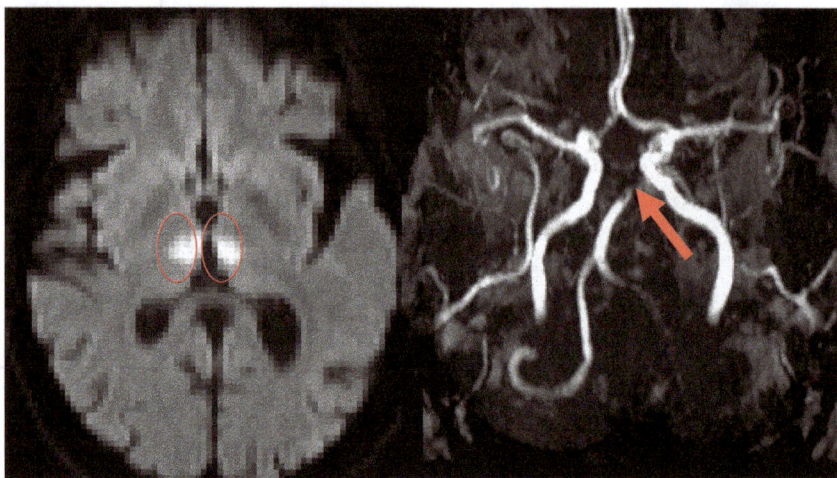

Fig. 6.1. Axial diffusion (A) demonstrates restricted diffusion within the bilateral thalami (*circle*) consistent with acute ischemia. Circle of Willis 3D MIP angiography (B) demonstrates complete occlusion of the distal basilar artery (*arrow*).

not, the patient should be admitted for evaluation of the etiology of the top of the basilar syndrome and for treatment of stroke risk factors.

Dr. Lee. In the modern neuroimaging era, patients can undergo a CT and sometimes an MRI within hours of presentation. If the studies are performed this acutely the structural imaging can be normal. A patient with an apparently unilateral and presumed "ischemic" third nerve palsy can have a normal CT and MRI. If bilateral ocular motor cranial neuropathy signs appear, then the differential diagnosis includes Bickerstaff's encephalitis, botulisum, Miller-Fisher variant, myasthenia gravis, Wernicke syndrome and Whipple's disease. The normal neuroimaging may give rise to a false sense of security, however, if DWI is not included in the study. The DWI might show bright signal (i.e. restricted diffusion) bilaterally due to "top of the basilar" thrombosis producing acute ischemia at the mesencephalic-thalamic junction, even though the initial structural studies are normal.

REFERENCES

Caplan LR. (1980) "Top of the basilar" syndrome. *Neurology* **30**:72–79.

Keane JR. (1990) The pretectal syndrome: 206 patients. *Neurology* **40**:684–690.

Pullicino P, Lincoff N, Truax BT. (2000) Abnormal vergence with upper brain stem infarcts. Pseudoabducens palsy. *Neurology* **55**:32–35.

7

Acute Unilateral Optic Neuropathy

CASE NO. 7

A 44-year-old white female presented in the ER complaining of gray vision in her left eye for three days. She also described some left eye pain that was worse with eye movement. She denied any other neurological symptoms. Past medical history was unremarkable.

On examination, her visual acuity was 20/20 OD and count fingers 6 feet OS. The pupillary examination showed 1.5 log unit afferent pupillary defect in the left eye. Ocular motility was full, but the patient noted some eye pain during movement. Slit lamp examination was unremarkable in each eye. Intraocular pressure was 16 mm Hg in each eye. Funduscopic examination showed a cup-to-disc ratio of 0.3 in each eye. The macula, vessels, and periphery were unremarkable.

Discussion

Dr. Brazis. The patient's clinical features are most consistent with optic neuritis (ON). Optic neuritis is an inflammatory or autoimmune disease process affecting the optic nerve, causing relatively acute impaired vision, and progressing over hours or days. Visual function is typically worse by one week, and the disease process is predominantly unilateral. Optic neuritis is more common in women (77%) and usually affects patients who are 20 to 50 years of age (mean age, 32 years). Pain, often induced or exacerbated by eye movement, accompanies visual loss in greater than 90% of patients. The optic disc is normal in approximately two-third of patients (retrobulbar optic neuritis) and swollen in one-third. Color vision is often affected more than visual acuity. Visual function is especially decreased in the central 20° of the visual field, with various abnormalities noted on perimetry. In the majority of patients, vision improves in the second or third week and is often normal by the fourth or fifth week. However, some patients do not improve to a functional level or at all.

The clinical features of a typical optic neuritis include:

- Acute, usually unilateral loss of vision

  o Visual acuity (variable visual loss 20/20 to NLP)
  o Visual field (variable optic nerve visual field defects)

- A relative afferent pupillary defect (RAPD) in unilateral or bilateral but asymmetric cases
- Periocular pain (90%), especially with eye movement
- Normal (65%) or swollen (35%) optic nerve head
- A young adult patient (<40 years) but ON may occur at any age
- Eventual visual improvement

  o Improvement over several weeks in most patients (90%) to normal or near normal visual acuity
  o 88% improve at least one Snellen line by day 15
  o 96% improve at least one line by day 30
  o Visual recovery may continue for months (up to 1 year)

- Patients may complain of residual deficits in contrast sensitivity, color vision, stereopsis, light-brightness, visual acuity, or visual field

Patients who meet these criteria are considered to have typical ON. Conversely, patients with the features listed below have atypical ON. Fundus features which should lead the examiner to consider alternate diagnosis to optic neuritis include lipid maculopathy ("macular star"), very severe disc edema with marked hemorrhages, cotton wools spots, vitreous cells, pale optic disc edema, retinal arteriolar narrowing, or retinopathy. Additional features suggesting an atypical ON for demyelination, include:

- Bilateral simultaneous onset of ON in an adult patient
- Lack of pain
- Severe headache (e.g. sphenoid sinusitis)
- Ocular findings suggestive of an inflammatory process

    1. Anterior uveitis
    2. Posterior chamber inflammation more than trace
    3. Macular exudate or star figure
    4. Retinal infiltrate or retinal inflammation

- Severe disc swelling
- Marked hemorrhages
- Lack of significant improvement of visual function or worsening of visual function after 30 days
- Lack of at least one line of visual acuity improvement within the first three weeks after onset of symptoms
- Age greater than 50 years
- Pre-existing diagnosis or evidence of other systemic condition
- Inflammatory (e.g. sarcoidosis, Wegener's granulomatosis, systemic lupus erythematosus)
- Infectious disease (e.g. Lyme disease, tuberculosis, human immuno-deficiency virus infection)
- Severe hypertension, diabetes, or other systemic vasculopathy
- Exquisitely steroid sensitive or steroid dependent optic neuropathy

In atypical cases, consideration should be made for a lumbar puncture and additional laboratory studies. The required evaluation depends on the history and examination, with specific attention to infectious or inflammatory etiologies. In addition, patients with inflammatory autoimmune ON often have progressive or recurrent, steroid responsive, or steroid dependent optic neuropathy.

The Optic Neuritis Treatment Trial (ONTT) was developed to evaluate the efficacy of corticosteroid treatment for acute ON and to investigate the relationship between ON and multiple sclerosis (MS).

The ONTT was sponsored by the National Eye Institute as a randomized, controlled clinical trial that enrolled 457 patients at 15 clinical centers in the United States between the years 1988 and 1991. The ONTT entry criteria included: patients between ages of 18 and 46 years; a relative afferent pupillary defect as well as a visual field defect in the affected eye; and examined within eight days of the onset of visual symptoms of a first attack of acute unilateral ON. Patients were excluded if they had previous episodes of ON in the affected eye; previous corticosteroid treatment for ON or MS; or systemic disease other than MS that might be a cause for the ON.

In the ONTT, all patients underwent testing for collagen vascular disease (antinuclear antibody [ANA]), serologic testing for syphilis (FTA-ABS), and a chest radiograph for sarcoidosis. Lumbar puncture was optional. An ANA antibody test was positive in a titer less than 1:320 in 13% of patients, and 1:320 or greater in 3% of them. Only one patient was eventually diagnosed with a collagen vascular disease. Visual and neurologic outcomes in these patients were no different from those of the other ONTT patients. The FTA-ABS was positive in six patients (1.3%) but none had syphilis. A chest radiograph did not reveal sarcoidosis in any patient. However, in a separate report, other authors described patient with isolated ON with a positive serology for Lyme disease. These authors recommended serologic testing for Lyme disease in patients with ON with or without the typical rash of erythema chronica migrans, who live in or have visited Lyme endemic areas. Cerebrospinal fluid (CSF) analysis was recommended for patients with positive serology and intravenous (IV) antibiotic therapy for unexplained pleocytosis. We do not order Lyme titers for patients with ON from non-endemic regions.

The evaluation recommendations of the ONTT study group for patients with typical acute ON include:

- **Laboratory testing**
  Chest radiograph, laboratory tests (e.g. syphilis serology, collagen vasacular disease studies, serum chemistries, complete blood

counts, etc.) and lumbar puncture are not necessary for typical ON but should be considered in atypical cases. (I also would consider Lyme serology in patients from endemic areas)

- **Neuroimaging**
  Neuroimaging studies in the ONTT disclosed an alternative etiology for visual loss in only one patient with a pituitary adenoma; a second patient had an ophthalmic artery aneurysm that was not detected on the initial magnetic resonance (MR) scan. The ONTT authors concluded that neuroimaging was of limited value in establishing the diagnosis of ON. MR imaging of the brain was felt to be a powerful predictor of multiple sclerosis (MS) and should be considered to assess risk of future events of MS and for treatment decision making.

Optic neuritis is the presenting feature in 25% of patients with multiple sclerosis (MS) and occurs at some stage of the disease in 73%. In a study of 60 New England Caucasians with isolated optic neuritis, the risk of clinical MS developing in 15 years was 69% for women and 33% for men. In another study, life-table analysis showed that 39% of patients with isolated optic neuritis progress to clinically-definite multiple sclerosis by 10 years of follow-up; 49% by 20 years; 54% by 30 years; and 60% by 40 years. This latter study did not note any difference in the risk of developing multiple sclerosis between men and women. In the Optic Neuritis Treatment Trial, the 5-year cumulative probability of clinically-definite MS was 30%. Brain MR scans performed at study entry was a strong predictor of the development of MS, with the 5-year risk of clinically-definite MS ranging from 16% in 202 patients with no MR lesions to 51% in 89 patients with three or more MR lesions. The Optic Neuritis Study Group further studied 388 patients who experienced acute optic neuritis and followed up prospectively for the development of multiple sclerosis. The 10-year risk of multiple sclerosis was 38%. Patients who had one or more typical lesions on the baseline magnetic resonance imaging (MRI) scan of the brain had a 56% risk; those with no lesions (191) had a 22% risk. In a final 15-year follow-up report of the ONTT, overall 50% of the patients converted to definite MS. The risk of developing MS was 25% when the baseline MRI was normal and 75% when MRI was abnormal (≥1 lesions). The risk of MS was significantly lower in those with a normal MRI who were male, had optic nerve swelling and atypical features of optic neuritis. The eventual degree of disability was not related to the number of baseline MRI lesions.

In the ONTT, the patients were randomly assigned to one of three treatment arms in the study:

- IV methylprednisolone sodium succinate (250 mg every 6 hours for 3 days) followed by oral prednisone (1 mg/kg daily for 11 days).
- Oral prednisone (1mg/kg daily for 14 days).
- Oral placebo for 14 days followed by a short oral taper.

The major conclusions of the ONTT related to treatment are summarized as follows:

- High-dose intravenous (IV) steroids followed by oral corticosteroids accelerated visual recovery (particularly with visual field defects; $p = 0.0001$) but provided no long-term benefit to vision.
- "Standard dose" oral prednisone alone did not improve the visual outcome, and was associated with an increased rate of new attacks of ON.
- IV followed by oral corticosteroids reduced the rate of development of clinically-definite MS (CDMS) during the first two years, particularly in patients with magnetic resonance (MR) signal abnormalities, but by three years, the treatment effect had subsided.
- MR findings were of prognostic significance for MS.
- Treatment was well tolerated with few major side effects (transient mood changes, sleep disturbances, dyspepsia, and weight gain occurred more commonly in the two steroid groups than in the placebo group. In the IV group, a psychotic depression developed in one patient and acute pancreatitis in another, both of which resolved without sequelae).

In a double-blind, randomized trial, 383 patients who had a first acute demyelinating event (optic neuritis, incomplete transverse myelitis, or a brainstem or cerebellar syndrome) were studied (CHAMPS study group). All had evidence of prior subclinical demyelination on MR imaging of the brain (two or more silent lesions of at least 3 mm in diameter thought characteristic of multiple sclerosis). The patients received either weekly intramuscular injections of 30 μg of interferon beta-1a (193 patients) or placebo (190 patients). The patients had received initial treatment with corticosteroids. During three years of follow-up, the cumulative probability of the development of clinically-definite multiple sclerosis was significantly lower in the interferon beta-1a group than in the placebo group (rate ratio, 0.56). At three years, the cumulative probability was 35% in the interferon beta-1a group and 50% in the placebo group. As compared with the patients in the placebo group, patients in the interferon beta-1a group had a relative reduction in the volume of brain lesions, fewer new lesions or enlarging lesions, and fewer gadolinium-enhancing lesions at 18 months. The authors concluded that initiating treatment with interferon beta-1a at the time of a first demyelinating is beneficial for patients with brain lesions on MR imaging that indicate high risk of clinically-definite multiple sclerosis.

The Early Treatment of Multiple Sclerosis (ETOMS) Study Group assessed the effect of interferon beta-1a on the occurrence of relapses in patients after first presentation with neurological events, these patients being at high risk of conversion to clinically-definite multiple sclerosis. Eligible patients had had a first episode of neurological dysfunction, suggesting multiple sclerosis within the previous three months and had strongly suggestive brain MRI findings. The patients were randomly assigned interferon beta-1a 22 μg or placebo subcutaneously once weekly for two years. Neurological and clinical assessments were done every six months and brain MRI every 12 months. 241 (78%) of 308 randomized patients received study treatment for two years; 278 (90%) remained in the study until termination. Fifty Seven (85%) of 67 who stopped therapy did so after conversion to clinically-definite multiple sclerosis. Fewer patients developed clinically-definite multiple sclerosis in the interferon group than in the placebo group (52/154 [34%] vs 69/154 [45%]). The time at which 30% of patients had converted to clinically-definite multiple sclerosis was 569 days in the interferon group and 252 in the placebo group. The annual relapse rates were 0·33 and 0·43, respectively. The number of new T2-weighted MRI lesions and the increase in lesion burden were significantly lower with active treatment. The authors concluded that interferon beta-1a treatment at an early stage of multiple sclerosis had significant positive effects on clinical and MRI outcomes.

Course. Our patient underwent an MRI study of the brain and orbits. Orbit MRI axial T1 post contrast with fat suppression demonstrates the abnormal left optic nerve enhancement (Fig. 7.1). Brain MRI

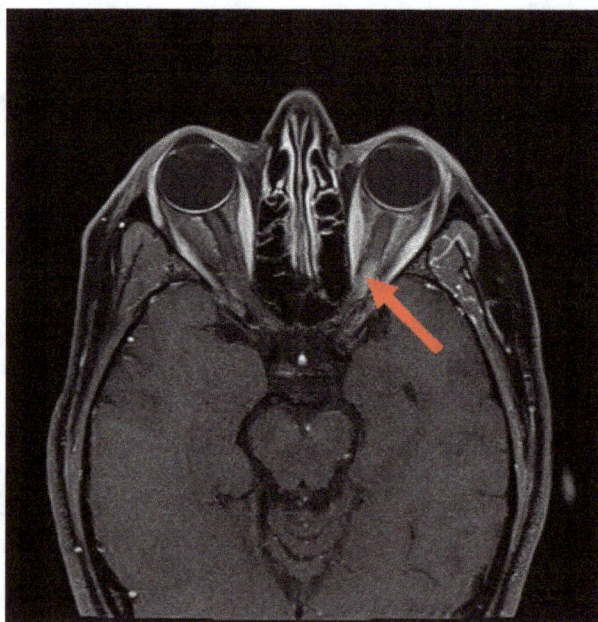

Fig. 7.1. Orbit MRI axial T1 post contrast with fat suppression demonstrates the abnormal left optic nerve enhancement (*arrow*).

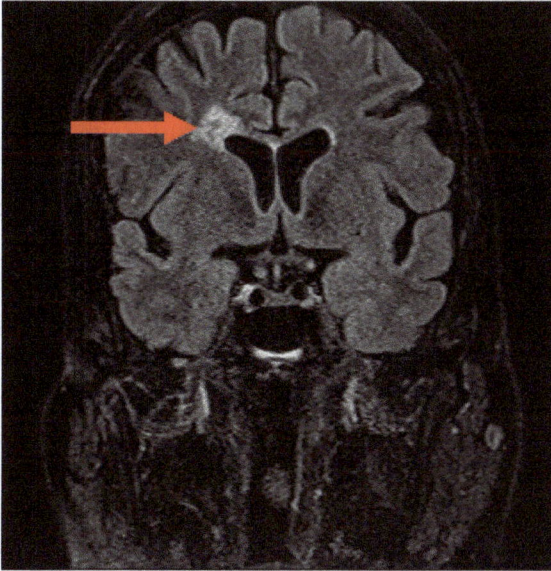

Fig. 7.2. Brain MRI coronal FLAIR demonstrates abnormal increased T2 signal in the right periventricular white matter (*arrow*) consistent with demyelinating disease. Other similar white matter lesions were seen in the periventricular white matter on other images.

coronal FLAIR imaging demonstrates abnormal increased T2 signal in the right periventricular white matter consistent with demyelinating disease (Fig. 7.2).

Because the patient is thought to be at risk for the development of multiple sclerosis in the future, she was offered intravenous corticosteroids to decrease or delay the risk of subsequent attacks. She was sent to a neurologist specializing in MS to discuss the use of immunomodulating therapies to decrease her subsequent risk of MS attacks and perhaps delay the onset of clinical MS.

Dr. Lee. Optic neuritis is a common cause of acute unilateral visual loss in a young patient. In patients with severe visual loss (e.g. 20/400 or worse), the clinician might make the mistake of skipping the formal visual field especially with other evidence for an optic neuropathy (e.g. RAPD, visual field defect, normal or hyperemic disc). The temptation is to make the clinical diagnosis of optic neuritis and schedule an outpatient MRI study. My recommended optic neuropathy protocol is a head and orbit study with T1 fat suppressed orbital views with gadolinium to look at the optic nerve, T1 axial post contrast brain to look for enhancing white matter lesions of active disease, and sagittal, coronal, and axial T2-weighted fluid attenuation inversion recovery (FLAIR) studies to look for demyelinating periventricular white matter lesions. If an imaging study is going to be deferred, the clinician should still test the fellow eye, even if asymptomatic, to look for evidence of not only optic neuropathy but also contralateral superotemporal visual field loss (i.e. the junctional scotoma) that might suggest an alternate diagnosis to optic neuritis such as a compressive lesion. Acutely pituitary apoplexy and ophthalmic artery aneurysm can both mimic a painful acute optic neuropathy but the junctional scotoma is definitely a red flag for a compressive rather than a demyelinating etiology. Likewise, patients who are elderly are unlikely to experience optic neuritis. The diagnosis of optic neuritis does occur in elderly patients but I always recommend cranial and orbital optic nerve directed neuroimaging. A retrobulbar acute painful optic neuropathy in an elderly patient is more likely to be posterior ischemic optic neuropathy from giant cell arteritis or a compressive lesion, including orbital apex fungal disease rather than demyelinating optic neuritis.

REFERENCES

CHAMPS Study Group. (2001) Interferon beta-1a for optic neuritis patients at high risk for multiple sclerosis. *Am J Ophthalmology* **132**:463–471.

Comi G and the Early Treatment of Multiple Sclerosis (ETOMS) Study Group. (2001) Effect of early interferon treatment on conversion to definite multiple sclerosis: a randomised study. *Lancet* **357**:1576–1582.

Jacobs LD, Beck RW, Simon JH, *et al.* (2000) Intramuscular interferon beta-1a therapy initiated during a first demyelinating event in multiple sclerosis. *New Eng J Med* **343**:898–904.

Jacobs L, Munschauer FE, Kaba SE. (1991) Clinical and magnetic resonance imaging in optic neuritis. *Neurology* **41**:15–19.

Optic Neuritis Study Group. (1991) The clinical profile of optic neuritis. Experience of the Optic Neuritis Treatment Trial. *Arch Ophthalmol* **109**:1673–1678.

Optic Neuritis Study Group. (1997) The 5-year risk of MS after optic neuritis. Experience of the Optic Neuritis Treatment Trial. *Neurology* **49**:1404–1413.

Optic Neuritis Study Group. (1997) Visual function 5 years after optic neuritis. Experience of the Optic Neuritis Treatment Trial. *Arch Ophthalmol* **115**:1545–1552.

Optic Neuritis Study Group. (2003) High- and low-risk profiles for the development of multiple sclerosis within 10 years after optic neuritis experience of the Optic Neuritis Treatment Trial. *Arch Ophthalmol* **121**:944–949.

Optic Neuritis Study Group. (2004) Long-term brain magnetic resonance imaging changes after optic neuritis in patients without clinically definite multiple sclerosis. *Arch Neurol* **61**:1538–1541.

Optic Neuritis Study Group. (2004) Visual function more than 10 years after optic neuritis: Experience of the optic neuritis treatment trial. *Am J Ophthalmol* **137**:77–83.

Optic Neuritis Study Group. (2004) Neurologic impairment 10 years after optic neuritis. *Arch Neurology* **6**:1386–1389.

Optic Neuritis Study Group. (2004) Multiple sclerosis risk after optic neuritis. Final Optic Neuritis Treatment Trial follow-up. *Arch Neurol* **65**:727–732.

Optic Neuritis Study Group. (2008) Visual function 15 years after optic neuritis: A final follow-up report from the Optic Neuritis Treatment Trial. *Ophthalmology* **115**:1079–1082.

Rizzo JF, Lessell S. (1998) Risk of developing multiple sclerosis after uncomplicated optic neuritis. A long-term prospective study. *Neurology* **38**:185–190.

8A

Acute Pupil Spared Third Nerve Palsy

CASE NO. 8A

A 66-year-old white male presented in the ER complaining of a headache for the past few days. On that day, he noticed that his right eyelid was drooping. He noted double vision since awakening in the morning, so he decided to seek medical attention. His past medical history was remarkable for diabetes mellitus controlled with diet/exercise, hypertension controlled with Lasix, and hypercholesterolemia controlled with statin therapy. His family history was unremarkable.

On examination, his visual acuity was 20/30 in each eye. Confrontation visual field was full in both eyes. Pupillary examination was normal without anisocoria or an afferent pupillary defect. Ocular motility was consistent with right third central nerve palsy (Figs. 8A.1 and 8A.2). Slit lamp examination showed a posterior chamber intraocular lens bilaterally and was otherwise unremarkable. Intraocular pressure was 14 mm Hg in each eye. Funduscopic examination was within normal limits in both eyes.

Discussion

Dr. Brazis. We divide third nerve palsy (TNP) into non-isolated and isolated TNP. The isolated TNP were defined as TNP without associated neurologic findings (e.g. headache, other cranial neuropathies). Patients with evidence for myasthenia gravis (e.g. variability, fatigue,

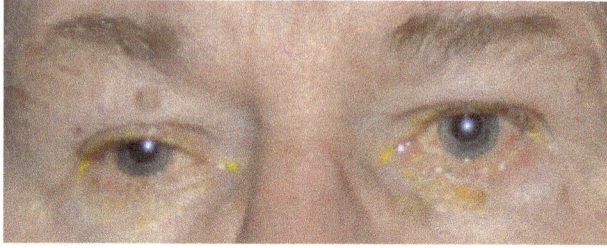

Fig. 8A.1. External photography showing partial right ptosis.

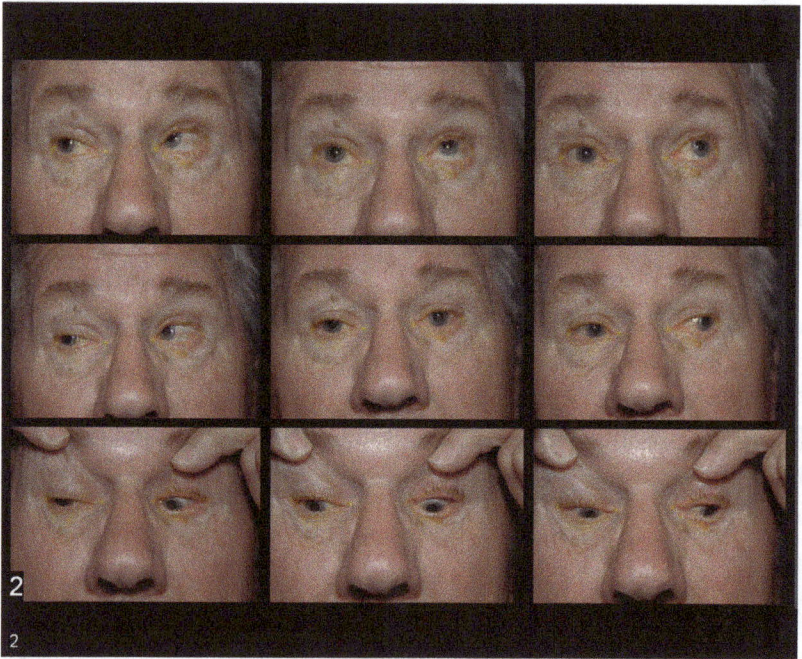

Fig. 8A.2. Ocular motility photography showing the right III nerve palsy.

Cogan's lid twitch sign, enhancement of ptosis) are not included in the isolated TNP group. We define six types of TNP:

Type 1: Non-isolated

TNP is considered non-isolated in the presence of the following features:

- Orbital disease (e.g. chemosis, proptosis, lid swelling, injection, and positive forced ductions)
- Evidence to suggest myasthenia gravis (e.g. fatiguability of the motility defect, Cogan's lid twitch sign, orbicularis oculi weakness)
- Multiple cranial nerve palsies (including bilateral TNP) or radiculopathy
- Brainstem signs (e.g. hemiplegia, cerebellar signs, other cranial nerve deficits)
- Systemic, infectious, or inflammatory risk factors for TNP (e.g. history of previous malignancy, giant cell arteritis, collagen vacular disease)
- Severe headache

Type 2: Traumatic TNP

Isolated unilateral TNP, which have a clearly established temporal relationship to significant previous head trauma and do not progress, are considered traumatic in origin. Patients with minor head trauma are not included.

Type 3: Congenital TNP

Patient born with an isolated TNP or noted to have a TNP within the first three months of life.

Type 4: Acquired, non-traumatic isolated TNP

- **Type 4A:** TNP with a normal pupillary sphincter with completely palsied extraocular muscles

- **Type 4B:** TNP with normal pupillary sphincter and incomplete palsied extraocular muscles
- **Type 4C:** TNP with subnormal pupillary sphincter dysfunction and partial or complete extraocular muscle palsies

Type 5: Progressive or unresolved TNP

Patients with TNP that worsen after the acute stage (greater than two weeks) or who develop new neurologic findings are considered to have progressive TNP. Patients without resolution of TNP after 12 to 16 weeks are considered unresolved.

Type 6: TNP with signs of aberrant regeneration

Non-isolated TNP should undergo neuroimaging, with attention to areas suggested topographically by the associated neurologic signs and symptoms. Appropriate investigations and neuroimaging studies are directed at the precise area of interest and this area determined by the associated localizing features with the TNP. In general, magnetic resonance (MR) imaging with and without gadolinium enhancement is the neuroimaging modality of choice for all these processes. Contrast-enhanced computerized tomography (CT) scanning with narrow (2 mm) collimation is reserved for those cases that cannot tolerate MR scan or in whom MR scan is contraindicated (e.g. pacemaker, claustrophobia, metallic clips in head, etc.) CT scanning is also the appropriate first choice neuroimaging study in patients being evaluated for acute head trauma or acute vascular events (infarction or hemorrhage). If there are clinical signs of a meningeal process, lumbar puncture should be performed.

The patient has an acquired, isolated, nontraumatic TNP. Acquired, nontraumatic isolated TNP may occur with lesions localized anywhere along the course of the third nerve from the fascicle to the orbit.

TNP with a normal pupillary sphincter and completely palsied extraocular muscles is almost never due to intracranial aneurysms. This type of TNP is most commonly caused by ischemia, especially associated with diabetes mellitus. Ischemic TNP may also occur with giant cell arteritis and systemic lupus erythematosus. Pupil-sparing third nerve palsy has also been reported with sildenafil citrate (Viagra) and similar agents and with cocaine use. Significant risk factors for ischemic oculomotor nerve palsies include diabetes, left ventricular hypertrophy, and elevated hematocrit. Obesity, hypertension, and smoking are also probable risk factors.

Ischemic lesions of the oculomotor nerve often spare the pupil because the lesion is confined to the core of the nerve and does not affect peripherally situated pupillomotor fibers. The pupil may, however, be involved in diabetic oculomotor palsies and diabetes may even cause a superior branch palsy of the oculomotor nerve. Pupil sparing has been documented in 62–86% of TNP due to ischemia. In a prospective study of 26 consecutive patients with diabetes-associated TNP, internal ophthalmoplegia occurred in 10 patients (38%). The size of anisocoria was 1 mm or less in most patients. Only two patients had anisocoria greater than 2.0 mm and it was never greater than 2.5 mm. No patient had a fully dilated unreactive pupil. The author concluded that pupil involvement in patients with diabetes-associated TNP occurs more often than has previously been recognized (14%–32% in other studies), although the degree of anisocoria in any one patient is usually I mm or less. Patients who have oculomotor nerve palsies with anisocoria of greater than 2.0 mm are considered outliers for the diagnosis of ischemia.

In a prospective study of 16 patients with ischemic third nerve palsies, 11 (69%) had progression of ophthalmoplegia with a median time between reported onset and peak severity of ophthalmoplegia of 10 days. All patients with an ischemic third nerve palsy will improve within 4 to 12 weeks of onset of symptoms.

Patients with an incomplete motor TNP with pupillary sparing require an MR scan to rule out a mass lesion. Pupil involvement is not diagnostic of aneurysmal compression, and up to 38% of presumed ischemic TNP involve the pupil.

Patients with a "relative pupil sparing" TNP should have MR imaging to rule out the possibility of a compressive lesion. Such patients should also have a CT scan if a subarachnoid hemorrhage is suspected and a subsequent cerebral angiogram if MR scan is negative because of the possibility of a cerebral aneurysm. In a small prospective study of 10 patients with "relative pupillary sparing" TNP, none of the patients demonstrated aneurysms. The authors suggested that the prevalence of aneurysm in patients with palsies of this type may be low enough to preclude routine angiography in the group. This report and subsequent recommendation was, however, based on an inadequate patient sample. In another report of 24 patients with relative pupil-sparing TNP, the authors found that 10 had nerve infarction, eight had parasellar tumors, two had intracavernous carotid aneurysms, one had leptomenigeal carcinomatosis one had Tolosa-Hunt syndrome, one had oculomotor neurilemmoma, and one had primary ocular neuromyotonia. Also, others have reported internal carotid, posterior communicating, and basilar artery aneurysms in isolated TNP with relative pupillary sparing. Thus, cerebral angiography may still be warranted if MR imaging is negative. Because up to 38% of patients with ischemic third nerve palsies have pupillary dysfunction, using these guidelines will yield a certain percentage of normal angiograms.

Complete external and internal third nerve palsies occurring in isolation are often due to compressive lesions or meningeal infiltration. A fully dilated and non-reactive pupil occurs in up to 71% of patients with aneurysmal compression and TNP. Aneurysms impair the pupil in 96% of TNP and the remaining 4% in which the pupil is spared have only partial TNP.

After having reviewed the literature on MRI/MRA, CT and CT angiogram (CTA), and catheter angiography in the management of the isolated TNP, we proposed the following guidelines:

- *Isolated complete or partial internal dysfunction (pupil dilated) with completely normal external function of the third nerve and no ptosis*

  The risk for aneurysm in this setting is minimal and neuroimaging for aneurysm is probably not required. The clinician should look for other etiologies for isolated pupil dysfunction (e.g. tonic pupil, pharmacologic, sphincter damage).

- *Partial external dysfunction TNP without internal dysfunction*

The risk for aneurysm in patients with partial TNP is moderate (up to 30% of cases). Unfortunately, the risk for an individual patient is not well defined because other etiologies may cause a partial external dysfunction TNP with a normal pupil. For example, patients who have clear myasthenia gravis do not require additional aneurysm evaluation. Other non-aneurysmal etiologies including neoplastic, demyelinating, infiltrative, and ischemic etiologies may also cause a partial TNP without pupil involvement and may require neuroimaging. If the TNP is due to aneurysm, the TNP usually progresses over time to a complete TNP with pupil involvement. Although there may not be internal dysfunction (pupil involvement) in a partial external dysfunction TNP, the term "pupil sparing" is probably not appropriate in this setting. That is, pupil involvement may occur over time in patients with partial TNP due to aneurysm with initially no internal dysfunction. Absence of pupil involvement early in the course of a partial TNP may be due to incomplete compression of the pupil fibers by the aneurysm. MRI with MRA or CTA in the acute setting is a reasonable screen in these cases. The patient should be followed clinically for progression or pupil-involvement in the first week. If the cranial MRI with MRA or CTA is negative and if the risk of angiography (e.g. elderly, severe cardiovascular disease, abnormal serum creatinine) is high, then observation alone is reasonable and the clinician should look for alternative etiologies for a partial external dysfunction TNP (e.g. myasthenia gravis). The clinician should still consider catheter angiography in these cases if the risk of aneurysm is higher than the risk of angiography (technically inadequate MRA, progression to complete TNP, pupil involvement). If a patient with a partial TNP has signs of meningeal irritation, other cranial nerve palsies, or signs of more diffuse meningeal involvement (e.g. radiculopathies), then a spinal tap to investigate infectious, inflammatory, or neoplastic meningitis should be performed. In case of presumed or suspected subarachnoid hemorrhage, a CT scan may be the preferred initial imaging study, followed by cerebral angiography.

- *Complete external dysfunction with completely normal internal function TNP*

  This clinical situation indicates a very low risk for aneurysm and the vasculopathic patient may be observed for improvement. The pupil should be re-examined within the first week. Patients who develop pupil involvement should be evaluated using the recommendations outlined under pupil-involving TNP. Vasculopathic risk factors, especially diabetes mellitus, hypertension, and increased cholesterol, should be sought and controlled. Patients over the age of 55 years, especially those with other symptoms suggestive of giant cell arteritis (e.g. headache, jaw or tongue claudication, polymyalgia rheumatica symptoms), should have a sedimentation rate determination. Temporal artery biopsy should be performed if the sedimentation rate is elevated or other systemic symptoms are present. If the patient has no vasculopathic risk factors, or if there is no improvement after 4–12 weeks, or if signs of aberrant regeneration develop, then cranial MRI with MRA or CTA should be performed. Evaluation for myasthenia gravis should be considered in painless, non-proptotic, pupil spared ophthalmoplegia, depending on the clinical situation.

- *Partial external dysfunction with partial internal dysfunction TNP*

  An initial cranial MRI with MRA (or CTA) is reasonable. If these studies are of excellent quality and negative, then the clinician should follow up on the patient for progression or complete internal dysfunction. The risk for aneurysm in this setting, however (even with a negative MRI/MRA), is uncertain. Clinicians should still consider catheter angiography if the risk of aneurysm in an individual patient is higher than the risk of angiography.

- *Complete external dysfunction with partial internal dysfunction TNP*

  The risk of aneurysm for complete external dysfunction with partial internal dysfunction (partial pupil or "relative pupil sparing") is also unknown but probably lower than for partial external dysfunction with or without partial internal dysfunction. The risk for aneurysm in this setting (even with a negative MRI/MRA or CTA) is uncertain. The clinician should consider catheter angiography if the risk of aneurysm is deemed higher than the risk of angiography.

- *Isolated complete internal dysfunction with partial or complete external dysfunction TNP*

This clinical situation has the highest risk for aneurysm (86% to 100% of aneurysmal TNP have pupil involvement). MRI with MRA or CTA of the head should be performed but even with negative neuroimaging there should be a strong consideration for catheter angiography.

- *Any patient with TNP and signs of subarachnoid hemorrhage*

The presence of SAH (on unenhanced CT scan or LP) essentially makes the issue of complete or incomplete TNP as well as application of the "rule of the pupil" moot. Unfortunately, most of the papers in the literature on aneurysm and TNP have included non-neurologically isolated cases including SAH. In general an initial CT scan (with consideration for a lumbar puncture) should be performed in patients with TNP and signs of SAH. The clinical picture of SAH (e.g. severe headache, meningismus, altered consciousness) can be mimicked by other intracranial etiologies such as pituitary apoplexy and most clinicians would consider a CT scan as an initial neuroimaging study prior to consideration of angiography. Patients with SAH on CT scan should probably undergo catheter angiography. Patients who cannot undergo a catheter angiogram (e.g. morbidly obese and unable to be placed on the angiography table) may have to undergo cranial CT and CTA alone prior to intervention. In other cases of SAH, special MR imaging parameters, including FLAIR MRI and MRA may be useful. Catheter angiography should be strongly considered even if the evaluations for SAH (e.g. CT, LP) are negative.

- *Patients who cannot undergo MRI or MRA*

  CT and CTA could be considered in selected cases especially if MRA is not available or in cases where MR is contraindicated (e.g. obesity, claustrophobia, pacemaker). Although CTA has some advantages over MRA (especially if the location of the aneurysm is known), the superior quality of MRI has compared to CT in evaluating the entire course of the third nerve makes the combination of MRI/MRA superior to CT/CTA as the screening study for TNP. There is insufficient evidence to determine if a combination of MRI and CTA would be superior to MRI/MRA in patients with TNP.

Dr. Lee. The "rule of the pupil" is that an isolated pupil-involved third nerve palsy should be considered to be an aneurysm of the posterior communicating artery until proven otherwise. A corollary to the "rule of the pupil" has been that an isolated pupil-spared complete third nerve palsy in a vasculopathic patient is unlikely to be an aneurysm. The "footnote" to these rules, however, states that the rules should not be applied to patients with partial third nerve palsy. In the past, the risk of catheter angiography (and its attendant morbidity up to 1% and possible mortality up to 0.1%) had to be weighed against the risk of missing an aneurysm. Modern noncatheter-based angiography, including CTA and MRA, have made it easier to proceed with less invasive and less risky imaging. A properly performed and interpreted CTA or MRA should detect 98% of aneurysms, producing a third nerve palsy. In my institution, CTA is our current initial procedure of choice but because an MRI with contrast is a superior imaging study for non-aneurysmal causes of third nerve palsy, the combination of CTA and cranial contrast MRI is probably superior to either study alone. The remaining 2% of missed sensitivity includes the differences in technique, imaging quality, and the neuroradiologist's interpretation of the study. Thus the experience of academic, tertiary referral center neuroradiologists spending extra time examining three-dimensional rotational images and source images from non-catheter angiogram may not be replicable or generalizable to all situations. Unfortunately, there is no pathognomonic set of clinical findings that can exclude aneurysm and most patients with a third nerve palsy will deserve consideration for some type of imaging study. I image third nerve palsies which are nonisolated, progressive, are partial, have any involvement of the pupil, or show aberrant regeneration. I do not think that anyone would fault the clinician for imaging even an isolated, pupil-spared, complete third nerve palsy in a vasculopathic patient but I generally at least offer observation for these cases, especially if the patient is already improving slightly by the time of my visit.

In my opinion, if the clinical suspicion for aneurysm remains high after CTA/MRA or if the noncatheter angiographic studies are insufficient to exclude aneurysm, then consideration should still be given for catheter angiography in all third nerve palsies, excluding perhaps the truly isolated, pupil-spared third nerve palsy in a vasculopath patient who improves over time.

Course. The patient underwent an outside MRI and MRA which were reviewed and were negative. A decision was made not to perform a CTA. The pain resolved within two weeks and the ptosis, and ophthalmoplegia all resolved after six weeks. The presumptive of an isolated ischemic third nerve palsy was made. The patient's internist optimized his blood pressure, blood sugar, and lipids.

8B

Acute Pupil Involved Third Nerve Palsy

CASE NO. 8B

A 52-year-old woman presented in the ER complaining of a sudden severe headache followed by emesis and photophobia. While she was being driven to the ER, she felt her left eyelid starting to close.

In the ER, her visual acuity was 20/20 OD and 20/30 OS. The left pupil was dilated and unreactive to light. There was limitation in adduction, elevation and depression of the left eye and complete ptosis OS (Figs. 8B.1 and 8B.2). The remainder of the eye exam was normal.

Dr. Lee. The clinical presentation of severe headache, nausea, vomiting, photophobia and signs of a third nerve palsy should be considered to be a ruptured aneurysm until proven otherwise. Although a complete exam is important in all patients in this setting, getting to a diagnosis quickly and then performing an imaging study might be life-saving. The motility findings are consistent with a third nerve palsy (Fig. 8B.2) and the pupil involvement should invoke the "rule of the pupil." The rule simply stated is that a pupil-involved third nerve palsy is an aneurysm of the posterior communicating artery-internal carotid artery junction until proven otherwise. Typically in this setting I would recommend starting with a noncontrast CT of the head to exclude hemorrhage (e.g. parenchymal, intraventricular, or subarachnoid bleed) and a contrast CT angiogram for aneurysm. If the noncontrast head CT shows subarachnoid hemorrhage or if the clinical exam is still highly suggestive of aneurysm, then catheter

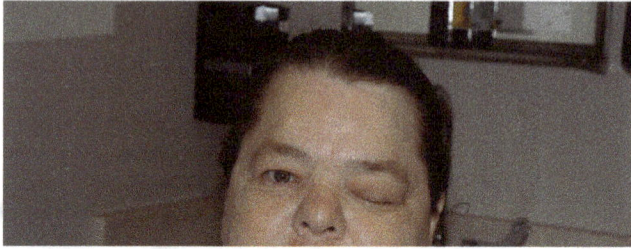

Fig. 8B.1. External photograph at presentation shows the complete left ptosis.

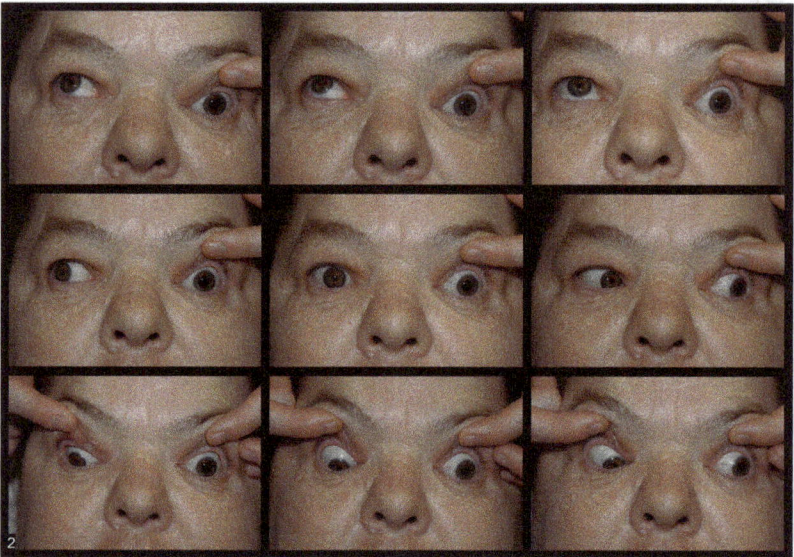

Fig. 8B.2. External photographs demonstrating a left third nerve palsy. Note normal abduction OS and there was intact intorsion on downgaze consistent with an intact fourth nerve function OS.

angiography might still be necessary even with a negative CTA. The use of CTA alone in this setting is highly dependent upon the skill of the interpreting neuroradiologist and the quality of the institution's CTA technology and the individual CTA images. In a patient with a third nerve palsy and no clinical or radiographic evidence for subarachnoid hemorrhage, then an MRI (MRA) is useful to exclude non-aneurysmal causes for third nerve palsy. Although in most centers a CTA is superior to an MRA for the detection of aneurysm. The MRI is superior to the CT scan for following the course of the third nerve for alternative etiologies other than aneurysm. The order of testing: CTA followed by MRI (MRA), or vice versa, is an individual institution's decision, especially as both techniques (CTA and MRA) continue to improve and have proponents on both sides.

Dr. Brazis. Acute third nerve palsy is a neuro-ophthalmogic emergency requiring immediate CT and CTA. Immediate evaluation by a neurosurgeon or endovascular aneurysm specialit is required. I agree with Dr. Lee's comments about the use of CTA vs MRA.

Course. The noncontrast CT scan showed intraventricular hemorrhage (Fig. 8B.3). The CT angiogram showed a left posterior communicating artery aneurysm (PCOM) and another asymptomatic right MCA aneurysm (Figs. 8B.4A, 8B.4B, and 8B.4C). The patient underwent diagnostic and therapeutic catheter angiography with endovascular coiling and obliteration of the aneurysm via interventional radiology.

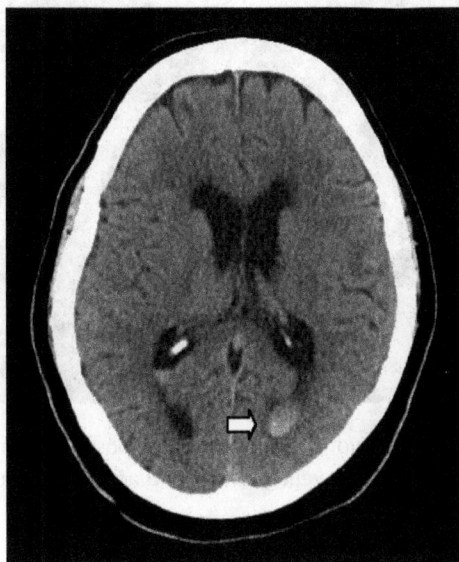

Fig. 8B.3. Noncontrast CT head shows hyperdensity consistent with blood in the ventricles (*arrow*).

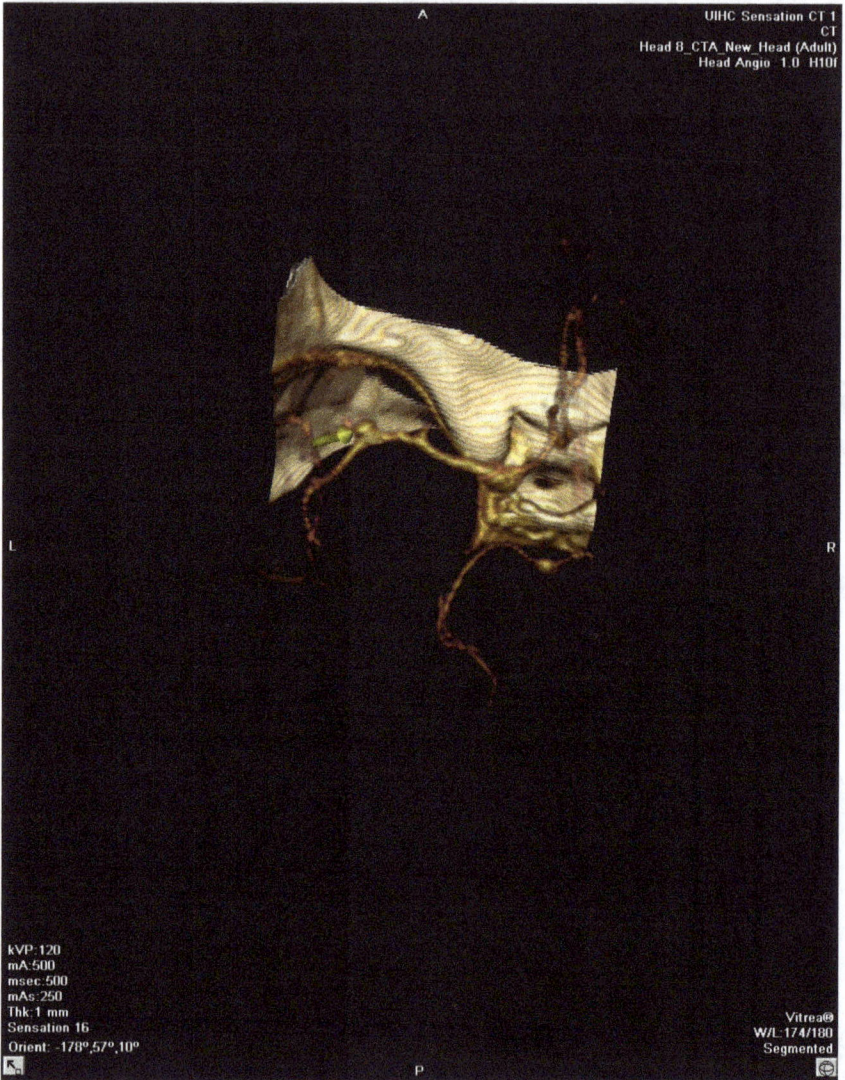

Fig. 8B.4. (A, B, C). A CT angiogram showing a left posterior communicating artery aneurysm (PCOM), labeled with yellow arrow and a right MCA aneurysm.

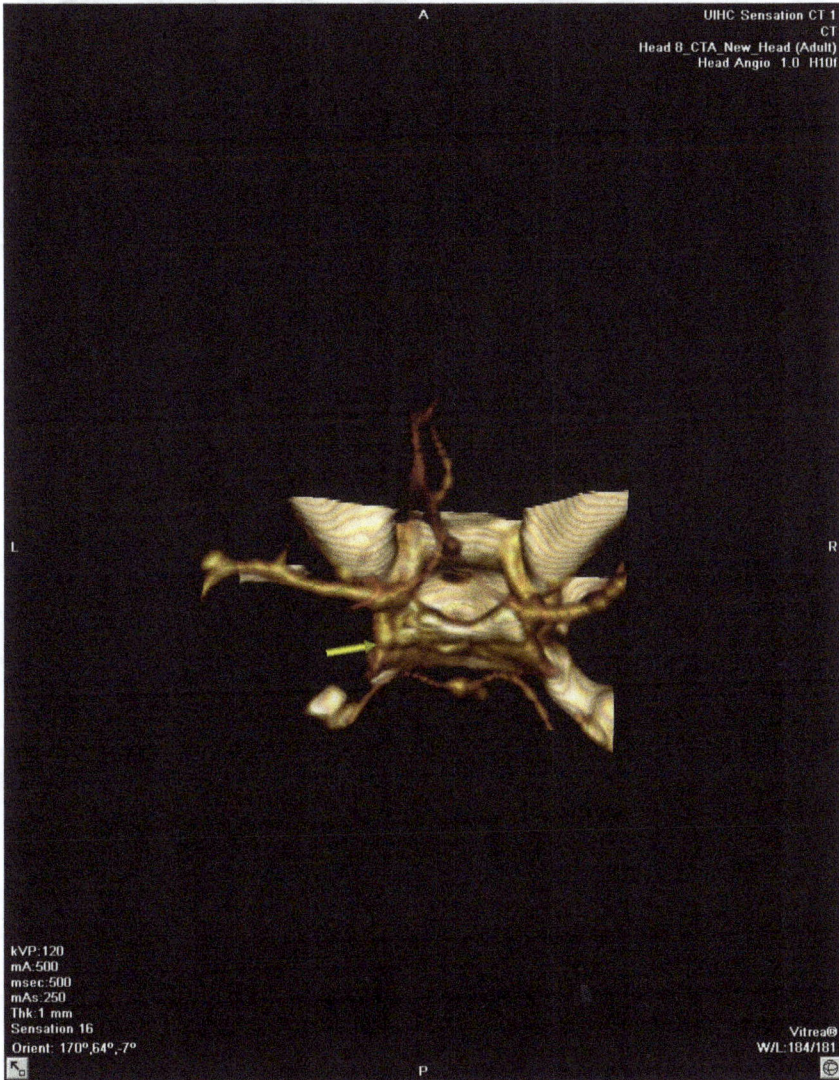

Fig. 8B.4. (*Continued*)

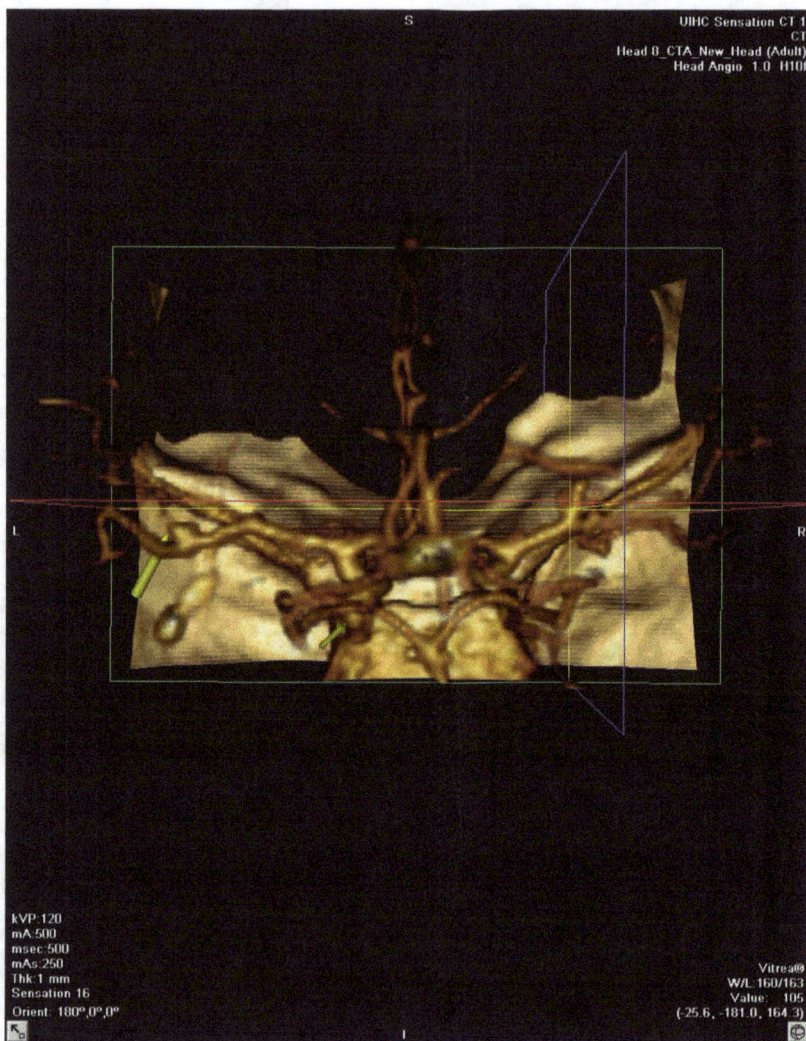

Fig. 8B.4. (*Continued*)

She was discharged from the hospital two weeks later. The third nerve palsy improved slowly over the next four months but did not resolve completely (Figs. 8B.5 and 8B.6). A follow-up diagnostic CTA showed complete obliteration of the aneurysm without recurrence. The second asymptomatic MCA aneurysm was treated one year later.

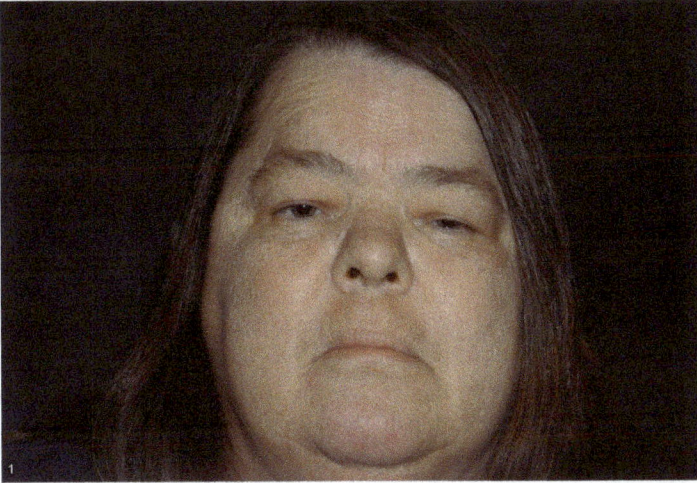

Fig. 8B.5. External photograph post endovascular coiling shows improving ptosis.

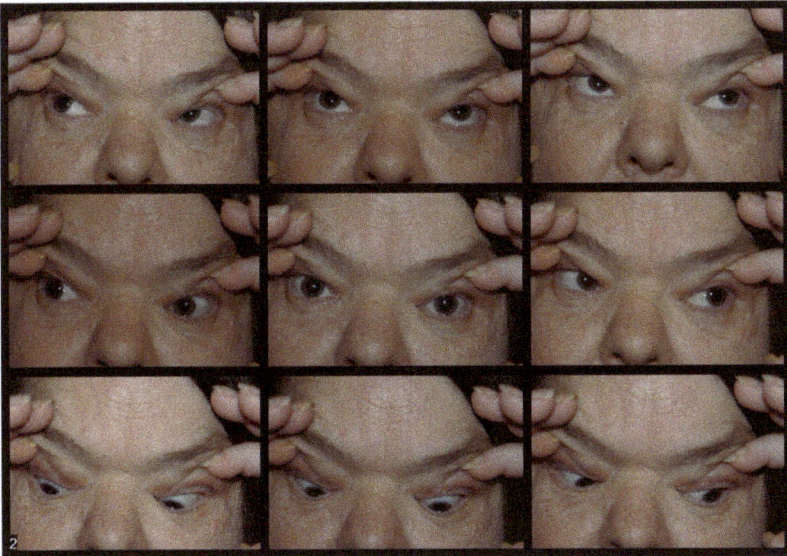

Fig. 8B.6. External photograph post coiling showing improved ophthalmoplegia.

REFERENCES

Cullom ME, Savino PJ, Sergott RC, Bosley TM. (1995) Relative pupillary sparing third nerve palsies. To angiogram or not? *J Neuro-ophthalmol* **15**:136–141.

Jacobson DM. (1998) Pupil involvement in patients with diabetes-associated oculomotor nerve palsy. *Arch Ophthalmol* **116**:723–727.

Jacobson DM. (2001) Relative pupil-sparing third nerve palsy: Etiology and clinnical vaiables predictive of a mass. *Neurology* **56**:797–798.

Jacobson DM, Broste SK. (1995) Early progression of ophthalmoplegia in patients with ischemic oculomotor nerve palsies. *Arch Ophthalmol* **113**:1535–1537.

Jacobson DM, McCanna TD, Layde PM. (1994) Risk factors for ischemic ocular motor nerve palsies. *Arch Ophthalmol* **112**:961–966.

Jacobson DM, Trobe JD. (1999) The emerging role of magnetic resonance angiography in the management of patients with third cranial nerve palsy. *Am J Ophthalmol* **128**:94–96.

Lee AG, Hayman LA, Brazis PW. (2002) The evaluation of isolated third nerve palsy revisited: An update on the evolving role of magnetic resonance, computed tomography, and catheter angiography. *Survey Ophthalmol* **47**:137–157.

Lee AG, Onan H, Brazis PW, Prager TC. (1999) An imaging guide to the evaluation of third cranial nerve palsies. *Strabismus* **7**:153–168.

9

Acute Proptosis with Red Eyes

CASE NO. 9

A 55-year-old white female presented in the ER complaining that her eyes have been bulging, the right more than the left, for the previous few months. She also related constant pain in both eyes. She denied any decrease in her vision. However, she stated that her eyes were always inflamed. Her past medical history was remarkable for rheumatoid arthritis under control with a nonsteroidal anti-inflammatory. Her family was remarkable for heart disease.

On examination, her visual acuity was 20/25 in each eye. The confrontation visual field was normal in both eyes. Ocular motility showed mild restriction of adduction and abduction in both eyes. Pupillary examination was normal in both eyes without an afferent pupillary defect. Slit lamp examination showed conjunctival hyperemia and was otherwise unremarkable. Hertel measurement was 24 and 20 (Figs. 9.1 and 9.2). Ophthalmoscopy was within normal limits.

Discussion

Dr. Brazis. The clinical features most likely suggest Graves' ophthalmopathy (GO). Graves' ophthalmopathy is characterized clinically by the following signs:

- Eyelid signs
  - Lid retraction (the most common clinical feature of GO)
  - Stare
  - Lid lag in downgaze

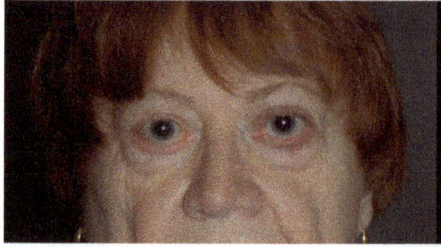

Fig. 9.1. External photography showing bilateral proptosis.

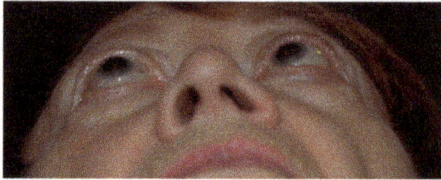

Fig. 9.2. External photography ("worm's eye view") showing proptosis OU.

- Exophthalmos
- Enlargement of extraocular muscles
- Increased orbi.tal fat volume
- Increased intraocular pressure
- Diplopia/ophthalmoplegia secondary to extraocular muscle inflammation or fibrosis
- Visual loss

  o Exposure keratopathy
  o Compressive optic neuropathy (CON) from extraocular muscle involvement in the orbital apex
  o Stretching of the optic nerve due to proptosis

- Signs and symptoms of orbital congestion

  o Due to proptosis with or without venous outflow obstruction
  o Conjunctival injection and chemosis
  o Eyelid and periorbital edema
  o Tearing, photophobia, and orbital discomfort

Patients without the typical features of GO should undergo further evaluation for other etiologies of these signs: proptosis (e.g. orbital tumor or pseudotumor), strabismus (e.g. myasthenia gravis), and/or lid retraction.

The differential diagnosis for Graves' ophthalmopathy includes orbital inflammatory pseudotumor characterized by the following features:

- Typically unilateral but may be bilateral
- Clinical signs of orbital mass effect and inflammation (e.g. proptosis, chemosis, pain, injection, ophthalmoplegia)
- Neuroimaging shows focal or diffuse inflammatory lesion
- Histopathology reveals a fibro-inflammatory lesion
- No other identifiable local or systemic causes

With orbital pseudotumor, when the inflammatory process is confined to one or multiple extraocular muscles, the process is referred to as orbital myositis, although some authors feel that orbital pseudotumor and orbital myositis may be distinct clinicotherapeutic entities. Patients present with acute or subacute orbital pain and diplopia. Findings include conjunctival chemosis and injection, ptosis, and proptosis. Angle-closure glaucoma may rarely occur. The process may be unilateral or bilateral and usually resolves with corticosteroid therapy or radiation therapy. The illness is often monophasic but recurrent episodes may occur. Characteristics associated with recurrences include male gender, lack of proptosis, eyelid retraction, horizontal extraocular muscle involvement, multiple or bilateral extraocular muscle involvement, muscle tendon sparing on neuroimaging, and lack of response to steroids or nonsteroidal anti-inflammatory agents. Orbital myositis may be associated with systemic diseases, such as Crohn's disease, celiac disease, Churg-Strauss syndrome, systemic lupus erythematosus, Whipple's disease, sarcoidosis, rheumatoid arthritis, linear scleroderma, and Wegener's granulomatosis. Recurrent orbital myositis may occasionally be familial and orbital myositis may occasionally be paraneoplastic. Orbital myositis may rarely mimic cluster headache and present with unilateral supraorbital pain, lacrimation, conjunctival hyperemia, nasal congestion, proptosis, and painful eye movements. Inflammatory orbital pseudotumor may occasionally extend beyond the orbit.

Neuroimaging in orbital myosisits reveals enlarged, irregular muscles usually with tendinous insertion involvement (as opposed to tendon sparing in thyroid ophthalmopathy). Intracranial extension of the inflammatory process is rare. The differential diagnosis of orbital pseudotumor is outlined below:

- Thyroid eye disease
- Orbital cellulitis (e.g. orbital apex syndrome) and infectious myositis

  o Bacterial

- Fungal

  o Aspergillosis
  o Mucormycosis
  o Bipolaris hawaiiensis
  o Actinomycosis

- Cysticercosis
- Trichinosis
- Gnathostomiasis
- Lyme disease
- Herpes zoster ophthalmicus
- Low flow dural-cavernous sinus fistula
- Neoplastic

  o Metastatic
  o Breast cancer (false "orbital pseudotumor" presentation)
  o Lymphoid hyperplasia
  o Non-Hodgkins lymphoma and Hodgkin's disease
  o Sinus histiocytosis with massive lymphadenopathy (Rosai-Dorfman disease)
  o Seminoma (bilateral nonspecific inflammatory or Graves-like orbitopathy not due to direct orbital metastasis)

- Infiltrative

  o Erdheim-Chester disease (idiopathic infiltration of the heart, lungs, retroperitoneum, bones, and other tissues by xanthomatous histiocytes and Touton giant cells.
  o Orbital amyloidosis

- Inflammatory

  o Sarcoidosis
  o Giant cell arteritis
  o Orbital polymyositis and giant cell myocarditis
  o Systemic inflammatory diseases (Wegener's granulomatosis, systemic lupus erythematosus)
  o Orbital inflammatory disease after pamidronate treatment for metastatic prostate cancer

With orbital inflammatory pseudotumor, biopsy may be required to exclude other diseases, except in pure myositic locations, in which the clinicopathologic picture is rather unique and surgical biopsy may damage the muscle, and in posterior locations, in which the optic nerve may be at risk during surgery.

Thyroid eye disease (thyroid orbitopathy, thyroid ophthalmopathy, or Graves' disease) is a disorder characterized clinically by lid retraction, lid lag in downward gaze, exophthalmos, diplopia (due to extraocular muscle inflammation or fibrosis), potential visual loss due to compressive optic neuropathy or corneal damage, and signs and symptoms of orbital congestion. The restrictive extraocular muscle involvement may be confirmed by impaired ocular motility during the forced duction test. The extraocular muscles predominantly affected include the inferior, medial, and superior rectus muscles and as the process causes muscle tightness or restriction, the diplopia is worse in the direction opposite to that of the involved muscle(s) action. Thus, hypertropia and esotropia are quite common in thyroid eye disease but exotropia is uncommon because the lateral rectus muscle is usually not markedly involved. In fact, if a patient with thyroid eye disease is noted to be exotropic, superimposed myasthenia gravis should be considered as there is an increased risk of myasthenia gravis in patients with thyroid eye disease.

Thyroid eye disease and orbital myositis may resemble each other clinically. Differential features are outlined below:

Orbital Myositis	Thyroid Eye Disease
• Male = Female	Females predominate
• Acute or subacute onset	Gradual onset
• Often severe orbital pain	Painless or "foreign body" sensation
• Motility problems early	Motility problems late
• Limited (paretic) ductions	Restrictive ductions
• No lid lag or retraction	Lid lag and retraction
• Neuroimaging of orbit	Neuroimaging of orbit
o Enlarged muscles irregular	Enlarged muscles often smooth
o Tendon spared	Tendon may be involved
o Often unilateral	Often bilateral

Orbital imaging, such as computed tomography (CT) and magnetic resonance (MR) scans, often demonstrate proptosis, extraocular muscle (EOM) enlargement sparing the tendons, increased orbital fat volume, and sometimes engorgement of the superior ophthalmic vein. MR imaging may be superior to CT scan in differentiating EOM edema (with elevated T2 relaxation times) from fibrosis. Serial short tau inversion recovery (STIR) sequence MR imaging findings may correlate with the clinical activity score. Ultrasonography of the orbit can also demonstrate EOM enlargement consistent with GO. MR imaging, however, is usually more costly than CT imaging.

Apical compression of the optic nerve in compression optic neuropathy (CON) may be seen on CT or MR imaging. Coronal as well as axial images are useful in the radiographic diagnosis of CON in GO. We recommend orbital imaging in patients with clinical evidence of an optic neuropathy and in cases where the diagnosis is uncertain or atypical features are present.

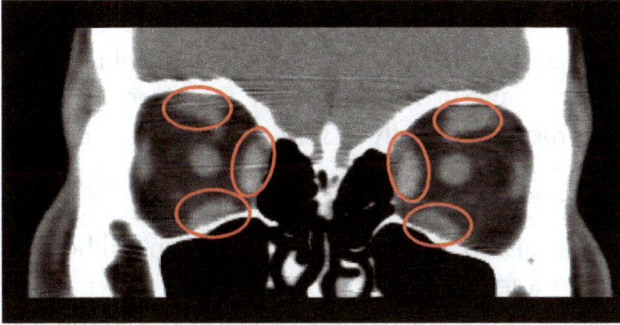

Fig. 9.3. Orbital coronal CT demonstrates the enlargement of the inferior rectus, superior rectus and medium rectus bilaterally (circles).

Course. The patient had a CT study of the brain and orbits. Orbital coronal CT demonstrates the enlargement of the inferior rectus, superior rectus and medium rectus bilaterally (Fig. 9.3).

Treatment of the underlying systemic thyroid abnormalities is the logical first step in the management of thyroid disease. The evidence is controversial regarding the effect of the degree of thyroid abnormality or the speed, type (e.g. medical or surgical), or completeness of systemic therapy on the incidence or severity of GO. Nevertheless, we recommend that systemic thyroid control be achieved and this may improve the signs and symptoms of GO. In a study of 90 patients with GO and hyperthyroidism in whom the severity of GO and thyroid function were assessed, patients were assigned to four groups with increasingly severe GO. More dysthyroid patients were in the groups with severe GO than in the other groups. Other uncontrolled studies, however, failed to show regression of GO after careful treatment of hyperthyroidism. Some authors believe that patients may experience worsening of GO after any systemic thyroid treatments (e.g. thyroid surgery, RAI, and neck radiotherapy for non-thyroidal neoplasms). The presumed mechanism for worsening GO is leakage of thyroid antigens and an increased level of circulating thyroid autoantibodies.

Several studies have shown that smoking is associated with worsening GO and we recommend discontinuing tobacco in all of our patients with GO. Smoking influences the course of GO during treatment in a dose-dependent manner. The response to treatment is delayed and considerably poorer in smokers. Insulin-dependent diabetes mellitus is also a risk factor for GO, and optic neuropathy occurs much more frequently (33.3%) in patients with GO and diabetes (and seems to have a worse prognosis) than in a total group of patients with GO (3.9%).

The natural history of the GO is variable and although most GO appears within a few months of the diagnosis of hyperthyroidism, it may have developed many months to years prior to the diagnosis, or many months to years after the onset of the systemic diagnosis of thyroid abnormality. Some patients never show clinical or laboratory evidence for systemic thyroid abnormalities (euthyroid GO). In many patients, GO is a self-limited disease that may not require any therapy and the disease often stabilizes within one to three years. Therefore, treatment is usually directed at short-term control of the inflammatory component of the disease (usually within the first 6 to 36 months); acute intervention for vision-threatening proptosis or CON; and long-term reconstructive management of lid retraction, strabismus, and proptosis.

Medical and other conservative therapy should generally precede consideration of surgical intervention. A logical stepwise approach to the surgical rehabilitation of GO is proposed in the following four stages:

1. Orbital decompression
2. Strabismus surgery
3. Lid margin repositioning surgery
4. Blepharoplasty.

The rationale for this sequential approach to GO is that orbital decompression often results in worsening, new, or changed extraocular muscle dysfunction as well as changes in lid position. Therefore, orbital decompression should in general precede strabismus and lid surgery in patients who require all three surgeries. Patients with CON should undergo treatment to preserve or improve vision.

A prospective, randomized, double-blind, placebo-controlled study of orbital radiotherapy for GO has been performed. The patients had symptomatic GO without optic neuropathy. Forty-two of 53 eligible consecutive patients were treated (20 Gy of external beam therapy to one orbit with sham therapy to other side followed in six months with reversal of the therapies). Every three months for one year, the authors measured the volume of the extraocular muscle and fat, proptosis, range or extraocular muscle motion, area of diplopia fields, and lid fissure width. No clinical statistically significant difference between the treated and untreated orbit was observed in any of the outcome measures at six months. At 12 months, muscle volume and proptosis improved slightly more in the orbit that was treated first. The authors concluded that in this group of patients they were unable to demonstrate any beneficial therapeutic effects. The usefulness of this study has been criticized, however, because of its broad patient inclusion criteria that lack rigor in controlling the issues of timing of therapy, the clinical variability in presentation of the patients, and multiple treatment methods used for individual patients. The same authors performed a three-year follow-up of 42 of their patients who had received orbital radiotherapy within six months of study entry. In this three-year uncontrolled follow-up phase, limited evidence for a clinically significant improvement was observed, which may have been the result of treatment or of natural remission. In either case, the changes were of little clinical significance. The authors concluded that because it is neither effective nor innocuous, radiotherapy does not seem to be indicated for treatment of mild to moderate ophthalmopathy.

The natural history of compressive optic neuropathy (CON) is poorly documented but presumably variable CON may be treated with systemic corticosteroids, orbital RT, or orbital surgical decompression. We recommend orbital decompression for proptosis in patients who have vision threatening exposure keratopathy or other significant symptoms (e.g. pain, pressure, severe exophthalmos) related to the proptosis.

Dr. Lee. Thyroid eye disease is typically not a difficult clinical diagnosis. The most common cause of unilateral or bilateral proptosis in adults is thyroid eye disease. I generally make the diagnosis clinically based on lid retraction, lid lag, proptosis, and ophthalmoplegia. Ultrasonography or orbital noncontrast CT scan are useful for confirmation of the clinical findings but are not mandatory if there is no doubt about the diagnosis and there is no evidence for thyroid optic neuropathy. I recommend an assessment of both activity and severity of disease. Active disease might benefit from immunosuppression versus inactive disease which might benefit from reconstructive or rehabilitative surgical intervention. Severity drives the decision making for treatment. In my opinion, mild disease is best treated conservatively as the natural history is typically one of improvement, spontaneously, over time. Compressive optic neuropathy (CON), however, generally requires treatment and it is reasonable to consider a short course of intravenous or oral steroids as a trial. Many patients have contraindications to steroids or may not be able to tolerate side effects and so my threshold for surgical treatment is low. Orbital decompression may be necessary for vision threatening compressive optic neuropathy. I recommend an orbital imaging study (generally noncontrast CT scan) prior to orbital decompression and for patients who seem to have markedly asymmetric or strictly unilateral findings. Control of the systemic thyroid status and discontinuation of smoking are important first line treatments for all degrees of thyroid eye disease.

REFERENCES

Bartley GB. (1995) Evolution and classification systems for Graves' ophthalmopathy. *Ophthalm Plast Reconstr Surg* **11**:229–237.

Bartley GB. (1994) The epidemiologic characteristics and clinical course of ophthalmopathy associated with autoimmune thyroid disease in Olmstead County, Minnesota. *Trans Am Ophthalmol Soc* **92**:477–588.

Bartley GB. (1996) The differential diagnosis and classification of eyelid retraction. *Ophthalmology* **103**:168–176.

Gorman CA, Garrity JA, Fatourechi V, *et al.* (2001) A prospective, randomized, double-blind, placebo-controlled study of orbital radiotherapy for Graves' ophthalmopathy. *Ophthalmology* **108**:1523–1534.

Gorman CA, Garrity JA, Fatourechi V, *et al.* (2002). The aftermath of orbital radio-therapy for Graves' ophthalmopathy. *Ophthalmology* **109**:2100–2107.

Kalmann R, Mourits MP. (1999) Diabetes mellitus: A risk factor in patients with Graves' orbitopathy. *Br J Ophthalmol* **83**:463–465.

Mannor GE, Rose GE, Moseley IF, Wright JE. (1997) Outcome of orbital myositis. Clinical features associated with recurrence. *Ophthalmology* **104**:409–414.

Mombaerts I, Goldschmeding R, Schlingemann RO, Koornneef L. (1996) What is orbital pseudotumor? *Surv Ophthalmol* **41**:66–78.

Mombaerts I, Koornneef L. (1997) Current status of treatment of orbital myositis. *Ophthalmology* **104**:402–408.

Prummel MF, Wiersinga WM, Mourits MP, *et al.* (1990) Effect of abnormal thyroid function on the severity of Graves' ophthalmopathy. *Arch Intern Med* **150**:1098–1101.

Prummel MF, Wiersinga WM. (1993) Smoking and risk of Graves' disease. *JAMA* **269**:479–482.

Shorr N, Seiff SR. (1986) The four stages of surgical rehabilitation of the patient with dysthyroid ophthalmopathy. *Ophthalmology* **93**:476–483.

10

Acute Visual Loss in a Leukemia Patient

CASE NO. 10

A 5-year-old white female with a history of acute lymphoblastic leukemia presented in the ER for re-evaluation of new onset visual change and gait disturbance. She finished her chemotherapy four months previously and has been in remission. Her parents noticed wider base gait over the past three days, and she started complaining of difficulty seeing early on the day she present in the ER.

On examination, her visual acuity was 20/260 in each eye. Ocular motility was full. Pupillary examination was normal without an afferent papillary defect. Slit lamp examination was unremarkable in both eyes. Ophthalmoscopy showed grade IV optic nerve edema bilaterally.

Discussion

Dr. Brazis. Leukemias are usually classified according to the predominate cell type, the degree of differentiation within the cell line, and whether the process is acute or chronic. Acute leukemia occurs most commonly in the first five years of life, predominates in boys, and is most often lymphocytic. Chronic leukemias occur in older patients, with chronic myelocytic leukemia usually developing in men 20 to 60 years of age and chronic lymphocytic leukemia affecting predominantly men between 45 and 60 years of age.

Neurologic complications of leukemia are caused by a variety of different processes. Neurologic injury may be caused by leukemia invasion of the leptomeninges, parenchyma, spinal cord, nerve roots, and peripheral nerves. Leukemia may also cause cerebrovascular disorders, both hemorrhagic and ischemic, through obstruction of intracranial vessels. Neurologic sequelae may result from various forms of treatment of the disease. Some neurologic disorders in patients with leukemia are paraneoplastic. In most cases, however, leukemic involvement of the CNS occurs from hematogenous spread or by direct invasion from adjacent affected bone marrow.

CNS leukemia is diagnosed by CSF analysis, requiring a minimum typically of greater than 5 white cells/μL in the presence of leukemic blast cells, using cytospin techniques. Since the advent of successful therapy of leukemia, the meninges have become the major site of leukemic relapse. With the advent of intrathecal chemotherapy and cranial irradiation as a routine CNS prophylaxis, the incidence of meningeal leukemia has declined to approximately 10%. Leptomeningeal infiltration can lead to infiltration of the intracranial portions of the optic nerve and chiasm. In most patients, visual loss may be slow and progressive, responding to radiation therapy, or extremely rapid.

Ocular findings are the initial manifestation in 3.6% of patients with acute childhood leukemia. Most ocular dysfunction in leukemia is related to direct invasion by neoplastic cells; however, hematologic abnormalities associated with leukemia and the sequela of hyperviscosity also contribute significantly to visual morbidity. The main sites of involvement are the orbit and adnexal tissues, the retina, the optic nerve, and the uveal tract.

Sophisticated chemotherapeutic regimens and the use of prophylactic CNS irradiation in the treatment of leukemia have made the prognosis for long-term survival better. Survivors may suffer leukemic invasion of the optic nerve during a relapse and should be considered a potentially treatable cause of visual loss. Clinical evidence of infiltration of the orbital portion of the optic nerve occurs primarily in children and adults with acute leukemia, especially those with the acute lymphocytic variety. Although active bone marrow disease and CNS involvement are usually present at the time that the infiltration becomes evident, optic nerve infiltration may be the first manifestation of recurrence or relapse.

Leukemic infiltration of the optic nerve may produce two distinct clinical patterns. In one pattern, the prelaminar and laminar portion of the optic nerve are infiltrated; in the second pattern, the infiltration is retrolaminar. Infiltration of the optic disk occurs less frequently than does retrolaminar infiltration.

When the optic disk is infiltrated, the appearance is that of a fluffy, whitish infiltrate within the substance of the disk. The infiltrate is usually associated with disc swelling and hemorrhage. In this setting the visual acuity is usually normal or only minimally reduced; however, if the infiltration, swelling, or hemorrhage extends to the macula, significant impairment of central vision may occur. Leukemic infiltrates of the retrolaminar portion of the optic nerve is associated with variable degree of optic disk swelling. The fluffy appearance that is characteristic of optic disk invasion is absent in such cases, but an associated retinopathy that includes evidence of both arterial and venous occlusion may be present. Leukemic infiltration of the retrolaminal portion of the optic nerve is usually associated with moderate to severe visual loss.

Because both patterns of leukemic infiltration of the optic nerve are associated with some degree of optic disk swelling, they must be differentiated from papilledema. In many cases, this is difficult, not only because in all three settings there is optic disk swelling associated with minimal if any visual loss, but also because it is not unusual for optic nerve infiltration to occur simultaneously with meningeal infiltration and increased intracranial pressure. For this reason, in all patients who present with optic disk swelling in the setting of leukemia, neuroimaging studies and a lumbar puncture must be performed. CT scanning and MRI imaging typically show generalized enlargement of the affected optic nerve often associated with a cuff of enhancement surrounding the nerve that represents leukemic cells.

Course. Brain MRI T1 images in our patient demonstrated enlargement of both optic nerves (Fig. 10.1, *left*). Brain MRI axial T1 post contrast imaging with fat suppression demonstrated abnormal enhancement of both optic nerves and chiasm (Fig. 10.1, *right*).

111

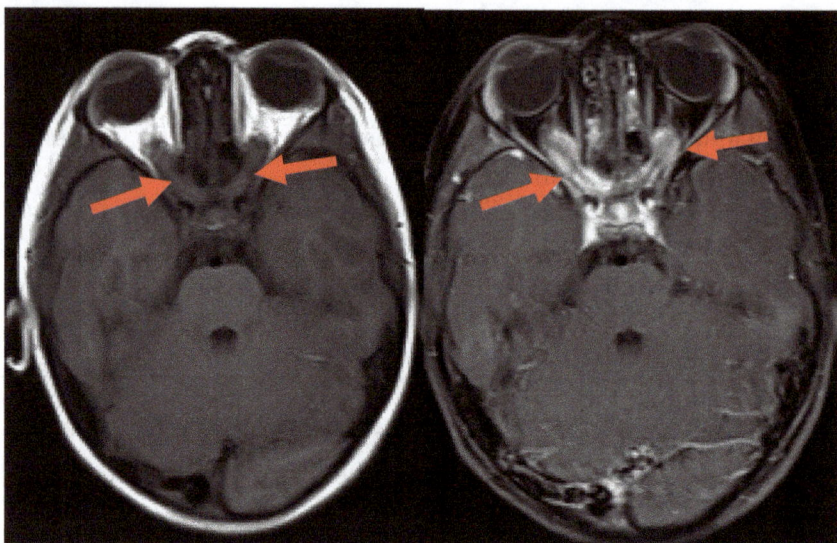

Fig. 10.1 (*left*): Brain MRI axial T1 without contrast demonstrates the enlargement of both optic nerves (*arrows*). (*right*): Brain MRI axial T1 post contrast with fat suppression demonstrates the abnormal enhancement of both optic nerves and chiasm (*arrows*).

Treatment of leukemia includes the use of chemotherapy, immunotherapy, and radiation therapy. The optimum treatment for infiltration of the optic nerves is usually prompt irradiation. Patients who receive about 2000 cGy to the posterior globe and orbit usually show a rapid resolution of the disk swelling and infiltration that may be accompanied by improvement of vision. Our patient's optic disk swelling resolved after chemotherapy (Fig. 10.2).

Dr. Lee. In general, patients who present with any neuro-ophthalmic complaint and a history of cancer should be presumed to have a recurrence of that cancer until proven otherwise. This is especially true for infiltrative neoplasms like leukemia. Leukemia can produce neuro-ophthalmic manifestations from the leukemia *per se*, from the direct treatments for leukemia (e.g. radiation or chemotherapy), or

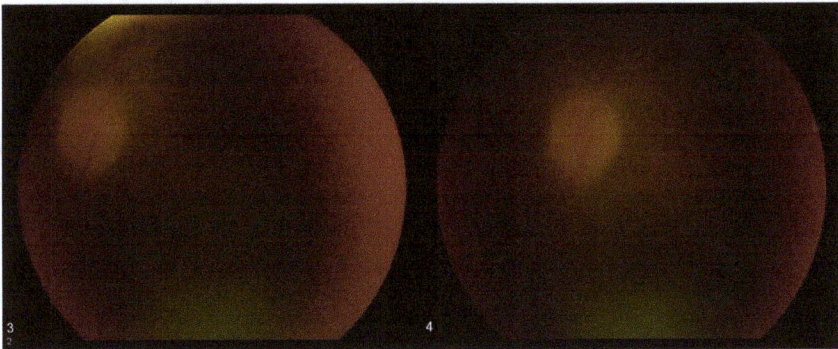

Fig. 10.2. Fundus photography showing the resolution of the optic nerve edema after chemotherapy.

from the side effects of treatment (e.g. immunosuppression, anemia, infection). Patients with an unexplained optic neuropathy who have underlying leukemia should generally undergo an aggressive evaluation (e.g. contrast enhanced cranial and orbital MRI with fat suppression and FLAIR sequences) to exclude CNS recurrence, and if negative, consideration for systemic evaluation for leukemic relapse and leukemic meningitis should be considered. The bottom line is that the clinician should be aware of leukemia relapse in patients with any neuro-ophthalmic signs or symptoms.

REFERENCES

Brown GC, Shields JA, Augsburger JJ, *et al.* (1981) Leukemic optic neuropathy. *Int Ophthalmol* **3**:111–116.

Camera A, Piccirello G, Cennamo G, *et al.* (1993) Optic nerve involvement in acute lymphoblastic leukemia. *Leuk Lymphoma* **11**:153–155.

Horton JC, Garcia EG, Becker EK. (1992) Magnetic resonance imaging of leukemic invasion of the optic nerve. *Arch Ophthalmol* **110**:1207–1208.

Kaikov Y. (1996) Optic nerve head infiltration and acute leukemia in children; An indication for emergency optic nerve radiation therapy. *Med Pediatr Oncol* **26**:101–104.

Modorati G, Calcagni M, Bandello F, *et al.* (1992) Bilateral involvement of the optic nerve in acute leukemia: Case report. *Ann Ottal Ocul* **98**:787–793.

Schocket LS, Massaro-Giordano M, Volpe NJ, Galetta SL. (2003) Bilateral optic nerve infiltration in central nervous system leukemia. *Am J Ophthalmol* **135**:94–96.

Shibasaki H, Hayasaka S, Noda S, *et al.* (1992) Radiotherapy resolved his leukemic involvement of the optic nerves. *Ann Ophthalmol* **24**:395–397.

Wallace RT, Shields JA, Shields CL, *et al.* (1991) Leukemic infiltration of the optic nerve. *Arch Ophthalmol* **109**:1027.

11

Acute Ophthalmoplegia After Vomiting

CASE NO. 11

A 20-year-old woman presents in the ER with recent onset blurred vision and diplopia. Her family has noted some confusion and mental status changes in her recently. She was one week post-partum and had suffered from hyperemesis gravidarum with persistent and recurrent vomiting, requiring intravenous fluids. Past medical history is significant for migraine and bipolar disorder. She admits to binge drinking alcohol 3–4 times a month but does not smoke cigarettes. She was not taking medications, however.

On examination in the ER, her visual acuity was 20/60 in each eye. She had mild light-near dissociation of both pupils with no anisocoria. In the primary position she had upbeat nystagmus which increased on upgaze and the amplitude and frequency of the nystagmus diminished on downgaze. There was superimposed horizontal jerk nystagmus in right and left gaze (Fig. 11.1). There was a small angle esotropia noted in the primary position and she had mild but symmetric upgaze restriction OU. The remainder of the eye exam was normal. A CT scan of the head in the ER was normal.

Dr. Lee. A patient with acute onset of mental status changes, nystagmus and diplopia in the ER and a negative cranial imaging for a posterior fossa lesion should be evaluated for Wernicke encephalopathy. Although classically Wernicke syndrome is associated with alcohol abuse, there may be an inaccurate or unknown or admitted prior history of alcohol use. The increasing use of bariatric

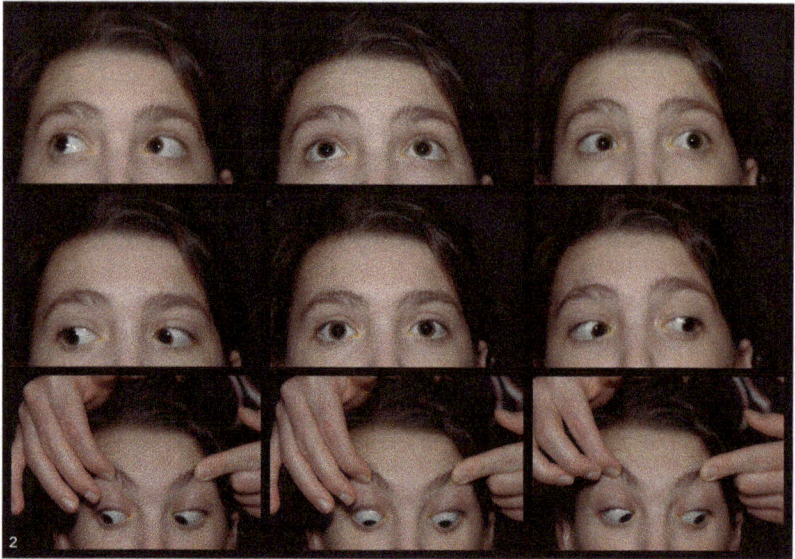

Fig. 11.1. In the primary position she had a small angel esotropia, and a slightly diminished upgaze bilaterally was noted. Not shown in this static photo is the upbeat nystagmus which increased on upgaze and diminished on downgaze with no null point. There was superimposed horizontal jerk nystagmus in the right and left gaze.

surgery in the US has increased the number of non-alcohol related cases of Wernicke that I have seen in my practice. In addition, malnutrition, use of total parenteral nutrition, and persistent vomiting (e.g. hyperemesis gravida) can produce the Wernicke syndrome. The triad includes ataxia, ophthalmoplegia or nystagmus and mental status changes, and may occur with any or all of the above. I would perform an MRI with contrast, but regardless of the imaging I tend to recommend giving empiric thiamine and magnesium to patients in the ER with acute unexplained ophthalmoplegia or acute nystagmus as the downside is minimal. I tend not to order the thiamine level and just treat empirically. In patients with unexplained ophthalmoplegia or nystagmus, imaging might show a brainstem lesion (e.g. neoplastic, infiltrative, traumatic, vascular, ischemic, demyelinating).

Dr. Brazis. In this patient, my major concern would be Wernicke's encephalopathy (WE). This is an organic global confusional ataxic condition usually thought of as seen in alcoholics and caused by thiamine deficiency. Patients with anorexia, severe weight loss of any cause, persistent vomiting, starvation of any cause, and patients who are desperately ill in intensive care settings are all at risk for development of WE. Stupor and coma are rarely seen in the initial phase of WE but untreated WE will progress to stupor, coma and death in a matter of days. The classic clinical triad of WE included ataxia, confusion and ophthalmoplegia. A newer operational definition of the syndrome emphasizes nutritional deficiency as the primary feature. Despite the importance placed on the ocular motor findings in both the classic and revised criteria for diagnosis, the incidence of these clinical findings is relatively low, occurring in only about a quarter to a third of patients studied at necropsy.

The visual problems seen with WE include bilateral, frequently asymmetric ocular motility disturbances and rarely acute nutritional optic neuropathy. Eye movement abnormalities include horizontal disturbances (e.g. gaze palsy, abduction paresis, vestibular paresis, internuclear ophthalmoplegia, horizontal nystagmus) and vertical disturbances (e.g. gaze evoked upbeat and/or downbeat nystagmus and skew deviation). Asymmetry of pupil size and impaired light response have also been reported in 19% of patients with WE, but this is the same incidence as simple anisocoria which occurs in 19% of the population at any given time.

The cause of WE is a deficiency of vitamin B1 (thiamine) which is a key coenzyme at three different points in intermediate carbohydrate metabolism. Depletion of thiamine and the subsequent stress of a glucose load may result in the relatively abrupt onset of WE. Blood levels of thiamine may be normal even in deficiency states, but blood transketolase levels reflect low thiamine levels more accurately. In this patient, however, we should not await the results of blood tests to initiate treatment. In addition, one should obtain serum magnesium levels (magnesium is a cofactor in glycolysis, which utilizes thiamine). If magnesium is low, it should be replaced when patients with WE are treated. Thiamine given in a patient

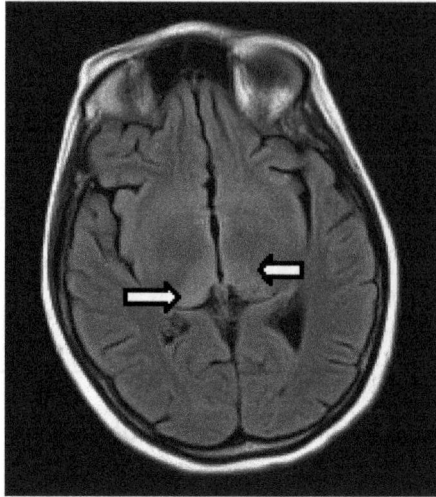

Fig. 11.2. Axial FLAIR sequence shows hyperintensity of the bilateral medial thalami (labeled with *arrow*).

with WE, when the magnesium level is low, will fail to reverse the clinical features of WE.

As far as neuroimaging in a patient is concerned, CT studies are of no help. MRI in patients with WE reveals a number of lesions best seen on FLAIR, T-2 and DWI sequences. High signals are found in medial thalamus, the hypothalamus, the mamillary bodies, in the periaqueductal region and surrounding the fourth ventricle. Other areas include the basal ganglia, cerebral cortex, pons and medulla. Imaging after treatment frequently shows generalized atrophy and volume loss throughout the entire brain.

The patient should receive the immediate administration of IV thiamine; 100 mg and $MgSO_4$ if serum levels are low. Oral thiamine, 50 mg daily, should be administered thereafter.

Course. MRI showed high signal intensity in bilateral thalami (Fig. 11.2). The patient was treated with empiric thiamine and magnesium and her nystagmus and diplopia resolved. The mental status improved and the patient was subsequently discharged.

REFERENCES

Cain D, Halliday GM, Kril JJ, Harper CG. (1997) Operational criteria for the classification of chronic alcoholics: Identification of Wernicke's encephalopathy. *J Neurol Neurosurg Psychiatry* **62**:51–60.

Foster D, Falah M, Kadom, *et al*. (2005) Wernicke encephalopathy after bariatric surgery: Losing more than just weight. *Neurology* **65**:1987.

Ghez C. (1969) Vestibular paresis: A clinical feature of Wernicke's disease. *J Neurol Neurosurg Psychiatry* **32**:134–139.

Harper CG, Giles M, Finlay-Jones R. (1986) Clinical signs in the Wernicke Korsakoff Complex: A retrospection analysis of 131 patients diagnosed at necropsy. *J Neurol Neurosurg Psychiatry* **49**:341–345.

Lam GL, Thompson HS, Corbett JJ. (1987) The prevalence of simple anisocoria. *Am J Ophthalmol* **104**:69–73.

Victor M, Adams KS, Collins GH. (1989) The Wernicke-Korsakoff Syndrome and Related Neurologic Disorders Due to Alcoholism and Malnutrition, 2nd ed. FA Davis, Philadelphia.

White ML, Zhang Y, Lee AG, *et al*. (2005) MRI imaging with diffusion weighted imaging in acute and chronic Wernicke encephalopathy. *AJNR* **26**:2306–2310.

12

Acute Anisocoria

CASE NO. 12

A 25-year-old female reports a difference in the size of her pupils after returning from a Caribbean cruise. The pupil was largest during the previous two days but appeared to have become slightly smaller. She denied any headache, ptosis, or diplopia and she had no other general or neurologic symptoms. She states that the left pupil is larger than her right pupil and that this was not present previously. Her past medical, surgical, family, and social history are non-contributory. The patient is a nurse and is concerned about having an "aneurysm."

On exam, her visual acuity was 20/20 OU. The right pupil measured 4 mm and was normally reactive to light. The left pupil measured 6.5 mm and was sluggishly reactive to light (Fig. 12.1). There was no light-near dissociation of the pupils. Both pupils were round. The slit lamp examination was normal OU. The intraocular pressure was normal OU. The motility exam was full and the eyes were straight in the primary position and the diagnostic positions of gaze. There was no ptosis. The fundus exam was normal OU.

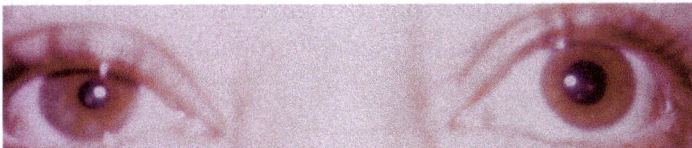

Fig. 12.1.

Dr. Lee. The evaluation of anisocoria is relatively straightforward and requires an assessment of the pupil light reaction and a measurement of the anisocoria in the light and the dark. In general, if the problem is strictly unilateral, then if the pupil reaction is impaired in one pupil, then that pupil is the problematic eye. If the pupil reaction to light is normal in each eye, then assessing the anisocoria in the light and in the dark helps to establish if the small pupil is not dilating (e.g. Horner syndrome) or if the larger pupil is not constricting properly. In this case, the left pupil is sluggishly reactive to light, indicating a problem with the efferent parasympathetic pupillary pathway or the iris on this side. If confronted with an abnormality in any one of the following three areas of the exam, namely the lid, pupil, or motility, then the clinician must always check to ensure a normal exam in the other two exam areas (I like to refer to this as "Savino's rule"). In this case of anisocoria with a larger pupil that is poorly reactive to light, the main concern is to exclude a third cranial nerve palsy. A careful assessment of the lid to exclude ptosis and an orthoptic evaluation in the primary and in the diagnostic positions of gaze, is critical to insure that the pupil finding is isolated.

An isolated dilated and poorly reactive pupil may be due to pharmacologic dilation, Adie tonic pupil, or local iris damage. The slit lamp examination is typically sufficient to eliminate local iris trauma or iris sphincter tear or anterior segment inflammation. Assessment for increased intraocular pressure (IOP) is useful as an elevated IOP can lead to damage to the iris muscle due to ischemia.

In patients with a fixed and dilated larger pupil and no other evidence for a third nerve palsy, topical testing with pilocarpine 1% might be useful to demonstrate that the pupil is pharmacologically blocked. Once the pharmacologic block starts to wear off, the diagnosis can be more difficult but the main concern is to exclude a third nerve palsy. If the patient has benign episodic pupillary dilation rather than pharmacologic blockade, it probably makes no difference in the end.

Dr. Brazis. As noted by Dr. Lee, patients with anisocoria and a poorly reactive pupil should be evaluated for an ipsilateral third nerve palsy.

A young patient with a thunderclap headache and a dilated pupil on one side has an aneurysm until proven otherwise. Check the ocular motility and lid for other signs of third nerve paresis. The pupil sign can be the first clue to an impending third nerve palsy and sub-arachnoid hemorrhage. Although an extra-axial lesion (e.g. unruptured intracranial aneurysm) compressing the third nerve may cause a dilated pupil in isolation (or with minimal ocular motor nerve paresis), in the absence of an extraocular motility deficit and/or ptosis, an isolated dilated pupil is usually not due to third nerve paresis. If there are signs of motility impairment suggesting a third nerve palsy, emergency neurologic evaluation and investigations in the patient is necessary.

Look at the pupil both grossly with a penlight and with slit lamp, looking for response to light, the near stimulus, and see if there is evidence of sector weakness, particularly in the more dilated pupil, as this could be a tonic (Adie) pupil. With a tonic pupil, there is usually mydriasis with a poor or absent reaction to light but a slow constriction to prolonged near effort (light-near dissociation). Redilation after constriction to near stimuli is slow and tonic. Segmental vermiform movements of the iris borders may be evident on slit lamp exam (due to sector palsy of other areas of the iris sphincter), and cholinergic supersensitivity of the denervated iris sphincter (constriction when 0.1% pilocarpine is instilled) may be demonstrated. Tonic pupils occur due to local damage to the ciliary ganglion or short ciliary nerves, as part of a widespread peripheral or autonomic neuropathy, or in otherwise healthy individuals (Adie tonic pupil syndrome). With time, ciliary muscle dysfunction tends to resolve, and the pupil becomes progressively miotic ("little old Adie's"). Some patients may have primary miotic Adie pupils without going through a mydriatic phase. There is a tendency for patients with unilateral Adie's syndrome to develop a tonic pupil in the opposite eye.

Damage to the iris due to ischemia, trauma, or an inflammatory process may cause mydriasis. The clinical characteristics suggesting abnormalities of the iris structure as a cause for mydriasis, include: no associated ptosis or ocular motility disturbance (vs third nerve palsy); the pupil being frequently irregular with tears in pupillary margin due to tears in iris sphincter (vs smooth margin in drug-related pupillary abnormalities); irregular contraction of the pupil to light; the possible eventual development of iris atrophy; and poor or no response of the pupil to 1% pilocarpine.

Mydriasis may be induced by the instillation of a parasympatheticolytic drug (e.g. atropine, scopolamine). For example, someone working with drugs like atropine or norepinephrine may get a little on the finger, and subsequently rub the eye. Or the mom who is demonstrating to her little child how easy it is to take an eye drop (atropine) may have inadvertently contaminated her fingers and transferred it to her own eye. Unilateral mydriasis may follow the use of transdermal scopolamine to prevent motion sickness, the accidental instillation into the eye of fluids from certain plants (e.g. jimsonweed) that contain belladonna and atropinelike alkaloids, and exposure to certain cosmetics and perfumes. A careful history is usually all that is required in patients with inadvertent or intentional (e.g. glaucoma medication, treatment with topical cycloplegics for uveitis) exposure to agents that may affect pupil size.

Nurses, physicians, and other healthcare workers are particularly prone to inadvertent or intentional exposure to pharmacological mydriatics. The pupil size of patients with pharmacologic sphincter blockade is often quite large (>8 mm), often on the order of 10 to 12 mm in diameter, which is much greater than the mydriasis usually seen in a typical third nerve palsy or tonic pupil syndromes. The pupils are evenly affected 360° (vs a tonic pupil) and smoothly affected around without irregularity (vs iris trauma). A solution of pilocarpine (1%) causes constriction in the case of a third nerve lesion but does not modify pupil size if the anisocoria is due to an atropinic drug or to iris damage. Remember, however, that some patients with Adie syndrome of recent onset may have a fixed dilated pupil that fails to constrict to even a strong solution of pilocarpine. Adrenergic pharmacologic mydriasis (e.g. phenylephrine) may be clinically distinguished by blanched conjunctival vessels, residual light reaction, and a retracted upper lid due to sympathetic stimulation of the upper lid retractor muscle. With adrenergic mydriasis, the pupil may react to bright light due to the working iris sphincter muscle which can overcome dilator spasm.

Course. The patient's pupil returned to normal after one day. She later recalled using a scopolamine patch for motion sickness on the cruise ship.

REFERENCES

Lee AG, Brazis PW. (2003) *Clinical Pathways in Neuro-Ophthalmology. An Evidence — Based Approach,* 2nd edn. Thieme, New York.

Thompson HS, Pilley SFJ. (1976) Unequal pupils: A flow chart for sorting out the anisocorias. *Sem Ophthalmol* **21**:45–48.

Thompson HS, Corbett JJ, Kline LB, *et al.* (1982) Pseudo-Horner's syndrome. *Arch Neurol* **39**:108–111.

13

Optic Disc Edema with a Macular Star Figure

CASE NO. 13

An 11-year-old boy presents with acute unilateral loss of vision OD. He had recently received a new kitten as a gift from his grandmother and he had been playing with the cat over the previous two weeks and received a few scratches. The past medical, surgical, family, and social history are unremarkable. He had mild flu-like symptoms one week prior to the visual loss but had no headache, lethargy, fever, lymphadenopathy or other neurologic symptoms or signs. The left eye was asymptomatic.

On exam, the patient's visual acuity was 20/200 OD and 20/20 OS. The pupils were 5 mm OU and both pupils were reactive to light but there was a right relative afferent pupillary defect. Goldmann visual field testing showed a dense central scotoma OD but was normal OS. Slit lamp biomicroscopy, motility, and intraocular pressure measurements were normal OU. The fundus exam was normal OS. The patient was seen by an outside eye doctor who noted optic disc edema OD and made the diagnosis of "optic neuritis" and told the patient's family that the boy might have "multiple sclerosis." A cranial MRI was performed and was normal. The patient was seen three weeks later in the eye clinic and had the fundus findings shown in Fig. 13.1.

Optic disc edema with a macular star (ODEMS) is a descriptive term encompassing a heterogeneous group of disorders. The condition has subsequently been called Leber's stellate maculopathy,

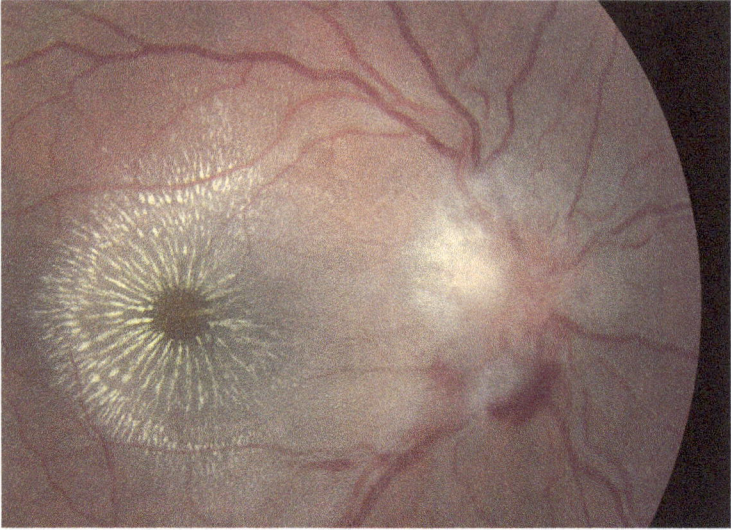

Fig. 13.1. Right eye fundus photograph shows marked disc edema, inferior peripapillary hemorrhage, and a full blown macular star figure.

Leber's idiopathic stellate neuroretinitis, or simply neuroretinitis. This syndrome is characterized by swelling of the optic disc, peripapillary and macular hard exudates which often occur in a star pattern, and, often, vitreous cells. Because the macular exudate likely results from primary optic nerve disease and not a true retinitis, we prefer the term idiopathic optic disc edema with a macular star (ODEMS) for idiopathic cases and use the term neuroretinitis when the optic disc swelling and a macular star are associated with retinitis, especially if an infectious cause is documented.

Patients are usually children or young adults, with the average age of onset of 20 to 40 years. Men and women are affected equally. Most cases are unilateral but bilateral involvement has been noted to occur in up to a third of the cases. Most patients present with acute unilateral loss of vision. The condition is often painless, but retrobulbar pain, pain on eye movement, or associated headache may occur. A nonspecific "viral" illness precedes or accompanies the visual loss in approximately half of the cases.

The clinical characteristics of ODEMS include:

- Age at onset: Childhood to young adult (6–50 years)
- Gender: Men = women
- Bilateral involvement: 5%–33%
- Pain: Occasional
- Antecedent viral illness: Approximately 50%
- Initial visual acuity: Variable (20/20 — light perception)
- Dyschromatopsia: Often prominent
- Visual field testing: Central, cecocentral, arcuate, or altitudinal defects; possible generalized constriction
- Relative afferent pupil defect present; but may be absent if bilateral involvement
- Optic disc swelling present with subsequent optic atrophy
- Macular star present but may take 1–2 weeks to develop
- Vitreous cells common (90%)

Optic disc edema is the earliest sign of ODEMS and may be severe. The disc edema tends to resolve over two weeks to two months but in some patients optic atrophy ensues. Optic disc edema is associated with leakage of disc capillaries with the fluid spreading from the disc through the outer plexiform layer of the retina. The serous component of the fluid accumulation in Henle's layer is reabsorbed, and the lipid precipitate forms a macular star. The macular star may be present at the onset of visual loss or may only be noted after one to two weeks following development of the disc edema. The macular star may even be observed only after the disc swelling has started to resolve. Patients with acute disc swelling with a normal macula should thus be re-examined within two weeks to investigate for the presence of a macular star, especially as it is of prognostic importance for the patient's subsequent risk of developing multiple sclerosis. Fluorescein angiography typically shows leakage from the optic disc in the mid- to late phases with abnormal permeability of the deep capillaries in the optic nerve head but no perifoveal leakage.

Most cases of ODEMS are "idiopathic" and thought to be the result of a nonspecific viral infection or some immune-mediated process.

In general, ODEMS is usually a benign, self-limited inflammatory process. However, a number of infectious agents and inflammatory diseases have been reported to cause ODEMS and neuroretinitis. It appears that syphilis, cat scratch disease, Lyme disease, and perhaps toxoplasmosis are the most common causes of ODEMS and neuroretinitis in cases where an etiologic agent can be identified. Infectious agents should be aggressively sought in cases of ODEMS and neuroretinitis because appropriate antibiotic treatment might be indicated. We recommended special emphasis on recent patient travel history (Lyme endemic areas), consumption of unpasteurized or uncooked foods (toxoplasmosis), sexually transmitted disease exposure (syphilis), and animal contacts (cat scratch).

There is no proven treatment for idiopathic ODEMS. Steroids have been used in some cases with unclear effect. If a specific infectious agent is discovered, than appropriate antibiotics should be considered. However, the data is limited.

Dr. Lee. I agree with Dr. Brazis that the term "neuroretinitis" should be reserved for infectious causes of ODEMS to avoid confusion. The main emergency considerations for optic disc edema with a macular star (ODEMS) are to exclude the mimics of infectious neuroretinitis. Patients with bilateral optic disc edema with a macular star figure might not have infectious neuroretinitis and instead might have disc edema from malignant hypertension or papilledema. I personally recommend considering imaging for bilateral cases especially if there is no vitreous cell seen or if the history is not compatible with an infectious exposure. Although cat scratch neuroretinitis is the most common etiology in my experience for the presentation of unilateral optic disc edema with a macular star figure, it is not clear from the evidence that treatment makes any difference in outcome. Nevertheless, I generally treat patients with serologic confirmation of Bartonella related neuroretinitis.

Course. *Bartonella henselae* IgM titers were positive and acute and convalescent IgG titers showed a titer elevation at 1:2048. The patient was treated with oral antibiotics and two months later had complete resolution of the optic disc edema and resolution of the macular star figure of exudate. The vision improved to 20/30 OD but there was residual retinal pigment epithelial atrophy in the macula OD.

REFERENCES

Brazis PW, Lee AG. (1996) Optic disk edema with a macular star. *Mayo Clin Proc* **71**:1162–1166.

Bhatti MT, Asif R, Bhatti LB. (2001) Macular star in neuroretinitis. *Arch Neurology* **58**:1008–1009.

Chrousos GA, Drack AV, Young M, *et al.* (1990) Neuroretinitis in cat scratch disease. *J Clin Neuroophthalmol* **10**:92–94.

14

Acute Transient Monocular Visual Loss

CASE NO. 14

A 44-year-old female judge presented with several episodes of transient monocular visual loss in the right eye. She described the event as occurring rapidly over seconds, lasting 10 minutes, and rising like a curtain over her vision. There was no precipitating or palliating factor and the events spontaneously arose and abated. The patient had no history of hypertension or diabetes but she was a heavy smoker (100 pack year history). She had no other neurologic signs or symptoms. She had a prior history of migraine headache in her twenties but no migraine visual aura. She saw an outside eye doctor and had a completely normal eye exam. She had no visual or other neurologic complaints at that visit. She denied any headache or pain. A diagnosis of "retinal migraine" was made and the patient was sent home.

The following day she developed several more episodes of amaurosis fugax OD. The patient called the eye doctor and was told to make an appointment with a neurologist for "migraine."

Dr. Lee. Transient monocular visual loss lasting minutes in an altitudinal (i.e. curtain over my vision) fashion should be considered to be ischemic until proven otherwise. The clinical dilemma is that although most cases of transient vision loss are benign (e.g. dry eye, corneal tear film disturbances), some cases are due to a potentially life-threatening cardioembolic source or visual threatening giant cell arteritis.

The history and exam provide key clues that should drive the triage and decision making for emergent versus routine evaluation and follow up. Isolated transient visual loss (TVL) is a different management issue from that of neurologically non-isolated TVL. Patients who have associated transient or residual hemispheric signs (hemisensory loss, hemiparesis, or aphasia) should be evaluated for stroke and consultation with our stroke neurology colleagues is advised. Likewise, if there is an acute and visible residual embolic event in the eye (e.g. branch or central retinal artery occlusion, Hollenhorst plaque), then I would defer to our stroke neurology colleagues for consideration for inpatient versus outpatient evaluation of cardioembolic sources (e.g. cardiac echo, carotid Doppler, laboratory studies).

The diagnosis of "retinal or ocular migraine" should be considered to be one of exclusion especially on the first event (which technically would not qualify for diagnosis by criteria). Many authors believe that this type of TVL is retinal vasospasm rather than migraine per se but this remains controversial. In this particular patient, however, the dangerous red flags suggesting an ischemic origin to the TVL include the duration of minutes, the onset in seconds, the altitudinal nature of the event, and the presence of vasculopathic risk factors.

The absence of the typical scintillation scotoma (e.g. positive visual phenomenon, jagged edge, colored lights, or fortification scotoma) or associated migraine headaches makes the diagnosis of migraine less likely even though this patient has a history for migraine.

Although giant cell arteritis would be unlikely in a 44-year-old patient, I would consider the diagnosis in all cases of TVL in an older patient and an erythrocyte sedimentation rate (ESR) and C-reactive protein as well as other investigations for giant cell arteritis might be warranted.

The bottom line in this case is that I am always hesitant to make a new diagnosis of "retinal migraine" in the absence of a classic history, multiple prior and stereotyped attacks without residual visual loss, and in an older patient. I am particularly concerned when the patient has other vasculopathic risk factors (older age, smoking, diabetes, hypertension, cardiac disease, or hypercoaguable state) and I typically defer to my colleagues in stroke neurology on the timing or need for admission for an inpatient evaluation. In patients with isolated TVL who have completely normal eye exams and who are not having repeated events, or in patients who have had multiple events without visual or neurologic sequelae over longer periods of time, I often concur with the outpatient ischemic work up. Patients with crescendo and recurrent events, with a visible embolus or with transient hemispheric signs, should probably be evaluated by a stroke neurologist on an urgent basis.

Dr. Brazis. Monocular TVL lasting 5 to 60 minutes (usually 2 to 30 minutes) is strongly suggestive of thromboembolic disease. Retinal emboli may arise from the aorta, carotid artery or the heart. Patients often describe the TVL as a veil or shade descending or ascending over a portion of their visual field. Other patients complain of patchy visual loss ("Swiss cheese" pattern) or peripheral constriction with central visual sparing. Some episodes of monocular TVL are accompanied by a sensation of color or other photopsias. Episodes of monocular TVL due to thromboembolic disease rarely last several hours.

Patients with thromboembolic disease may demonstrate emboli within the retinal vessels. Emboli may be composed of clotted blood, fibrin, platelets, atheromatous tissue, white cells, calcium, infectious organisms (septic emboli), air, fat, tumor cells, amniotic fluid, or foreign materials (e.g. talc, artificial valve material, catheters, silicone, cornstarch, mercury, corticosteroids). The most common types of emboli seen in atherosclerotic disease of the aorta/carotid arteries or cardiac disease include the following:

- Cholesterol emboli (Hollenhorst plaques) are bright, glistening, yellow or copper-colored fragments, most often seen in peripheral arterioles in the temporal fundus. These emboli most often arise from atheromatous plaques in the aorta or carotid bifurcation.
- Platelet-fibrin emboli are dull, white, gray, often elongated, and subject to fragmentation and distal movement. These emboli most often lodge at bifurcations of retinal vessels and arise from the

walls of atherosclerotic arteries or from the heart, especially from heart valves. They may also be seen in coagulopathies.

• Calcific emboli tend to be large, ovoid or rectangular, and chalky-white. These emboli often occur over or adjacent to the optic disc. They usually arise from cardiac (aortic or mitral) valves and less often from the aorta or carotid artery. Unlike cholesterol emboli, which often disappear in a few days, calcific emboli may remain permanently visible.

TVL may also occur from ocular hypoperfusion rather than embolization. In some patients, monocular TVL may occur when the patient is exposed to bright light. These patients usually have severe, ipsilateral carotid occlusive disease. Bilateral, simultaneous TVL induced by exposure to bright light may rarely occur with bilateral severe carotid stenosis or occlusion. The light-induced TVL probably reflects the inability of a borderline ocular circulation to sustain the increased retinal metabolic activity associated with light exposure. Alternating transient visual loss to bright light has also been described with giant cell arteritis.

TVL may also occur with carotid artery dissection. In a review of the clinical features of 146 patients with extracranial carotid artery dissection, 41 patients (28%) had monocular TVL. The TVL was painful in 31 cases, associated with a Horner's syndrome in 13 cases, and described as "scintillations" or "flashing lights" (often related to postural changes suggesting choroidal hypoperfusion) in 23 cases. Two of 23 patients with spontaneous carotid artery dissection experienced transient monocular blindness; in one of these patients, episodes were provoked by sitting up from a supine position.

Postprandial transient visual loss has also been described. It is proposed that postprandial visual loss may be a symptom of critical carotid stenosis, with retinal and choroidal hypoperfusion probably caused by a combination of mesenteric steal, decreased cardiac output, and abnormal vasomotor control.

TVL lasting 10 to 40 minutes may occur with central retinal vein occlusion or with impending central retinal vein occlusion. Venous stasis retinopathy (i.e. hypotensive retinopathy), associated with severe carotid or ophthalmic artery occlusive disease, may also be associated with TVL. This syndrome is characterized by visual loss and ischemic retinal infarction often accompanied by signs of ciliary artery obstruction, pallor of the disc, and hypotony. Venous stasis retinopathy may simulate Purtscher's retinopathy (multifocal areas of ischemia) and be associated with a variety of fundus pictures:

- Minimal or no ophthalmoscopic changes in some patients with monocular TVL.
- Few widely scattered blot and dot hemorrhages and mild dilation of retinal veins (venous stasis retinopathy), usually in patients with minimal visual complaints.
- Dilation of the retinal arterial tree, dilation of the retinal veins, and cotton-wool patches.
- Retinal capillary changes, including microaneurysms, cystoid macular edema, and angiographic evidence of areas of capillary nonperfusion that may be confined to the areas along the horizontal raphe.
- Larger areas of peripheral capillary nonperfusion, retinal neovascularization, and hemorrhage.
- Any degree of branch retinal vein occlusion, branch retinal artery occlusion, and central retinal artery occlusion.
- Ischemic optic neuropathy.
- Fluorescein angiography showing diffuse retinal capillary telangiectasia, delayed retinal artery circulation time, late staining of the disc, and aggregations of microaneurysms around the preequatorial zone mimicking idiopathic juxtafoveal retinal telangiectasia.
- Any of the above associated with panuveitis, neovascular glaucoma, and a rapidly progressing cataract (ocular ischemic syndrome).

Giant cell arteritis may produce attacks of TVL lasting minutes to hours indistinguishable from those produced by atheromatous disease. TVL probably results from intermittent inflammatory occlusion of the ophthalmic, posterior ciliary, or central retinal arteries. A postural form of TVL has been described in giant cell arteritis and a tenuous optic disc perfusion. Alternating monocular TVL may occur with GCA and may be induced by bright light.

TVL may also occur in association with antiphospholipid antibodies, hyperviscosity and hypercoaguable states, polycythemia vera, systemic lupus erythematosus, and hepatitis C associated type II cryoglobulinemia-mediated systemic vasculitis with mononeuritis multiplex. Arteriovenous malformations may divert blood flow from or reduce blood flow in the ophthalmic artery (ophthalmic steal syndrome). The TVL may alternate from eye to eye.

Vasospasm, especially associated with migraine, may also produce TVL without any of the visual phenomena typically seen during a migraine attack. Vasospasm of the retinal vessels has been documented by ophthalmoscopy during some attacks of monocular TVL. TVL, likely due to vasospasm and migraine, may be induced by exercise or sexual intercourse.

Intermittent angle closure glaucoma may also cause brief episodes of monocular TVL that are usually, but not always, associated with ipsilateral eye pain and occasionally simultaneous dilation of the pupil. Exercised-induced visual disturbances may also occur during attacks of pigmentary glaucoma. Episodes of monocular TVL lasting two to three minutes, induced by changes in posture, have been described following scleral buckle procedure, likely due to intermittent obstruction of the central retinal artery blood flow by the encircling element. Finally, TVL may also be associated with the congenital anomalies, peripapillary staphyloma and morning glory syndrome. Episodes of TVL with these anomalies may last 15 to 20 seconds or up to 20 minutes, the latter mimicking TVL with thromboembolic disease. The episodes of TVL in peripapillary staphyloma may be associated with intermittent dilation of the retinal veins and may be orthostatic.

Patients with monocular TVL, lasting minutes, associated with visible retinal emboli need to be evaluated for carotid and aortic vascular disease and cardiac valvular disease. Stroke risk factors (e.g. smoking, hypertension, diabetes mellitus, hyperlipidemia, etc.) should be evaluated and controlled. Studies to evaluate the carotid arteries include carotid Doppler and ultrasound. Some patients may require MR angiography and conventional angiography. Cardiac investigations include transthoracic and transesophageal echocardiography and cardiac MR imaging.

If no thromboembolic source for the episodes of TVL is documented, then further studies should be considered. These include MR imaging of the brain with MR angiography to investigate for possible brain ischemia, or less likely, a vascular malformation. Laboratory studies, including sedimentation rate, complete blood count, antiphospholipid antibodies, antinuclear antibodies, collagen vascular disease profile, and studies to investigate the presence of dysproteinemia.

Young patients (<45 years old) with monocular TVL are unlikely to have significant occlusive carotid disease (other than carotid dissection). A cardiac embolic source as well as a vasculitis or coagulopathy must be sought. As noted above, monocular TVL in younger patients has a more benign clinical course than that found in an older population and migraine is a likely cause of many episodes. Calcium channel blockers (e.g. verapamil or nifedipine), if not otherwise contraindicated, may be considered in some of these patients to reduce the frequency of episodes of TVL.

Finally, all patients with monocular TVL lasting minutes should have a complete ophthalmoscopic examination to investigate for such conditions as intermittent angle closure glaucoma, morning glory syndrome, and peripapillary staphyloma. Spontaneous anterior chamber hemorrhage (hyphema) should also be considered, especially in patients with associated erythropsia and in those who have undergone cataract extraction.

Episodes of monocular TVL lasting hours are rare. However, such spells may occur with thromboembolic disease, as a postprandial phenomenon associated with critical carotid stenosis, and with migraine. Monocular TVL lasting hours may be a symptom of impending central retinal vein occlusion.

Course. The following day, however, she developed weakness of the left arm. She was seen in the Emergency Room and a CT scan and subsequent cranial MR scan showed a right frontotemporal parietal infarct (Figs. 14.1A and 14.1B). An MRA showed a severe narrowing and hypoplastic right internal carotid artery A1 segment. The patient then

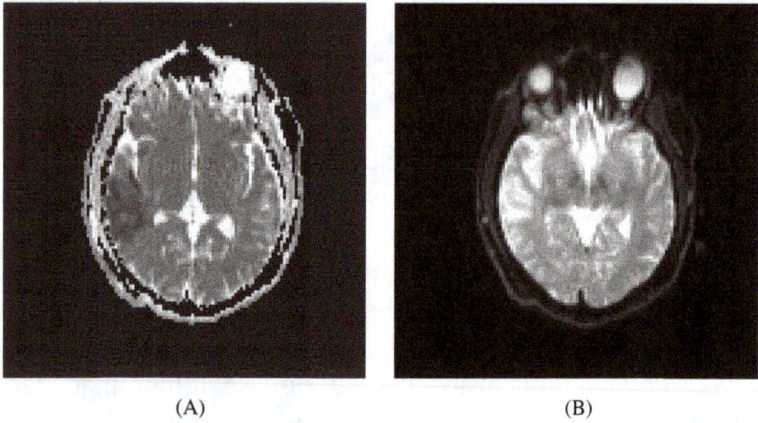

(A)   (B)

Fig. 14.1 (A, B) Diffusion restriction and ADI images show changes suspicious for a right frontoparietal infarct.

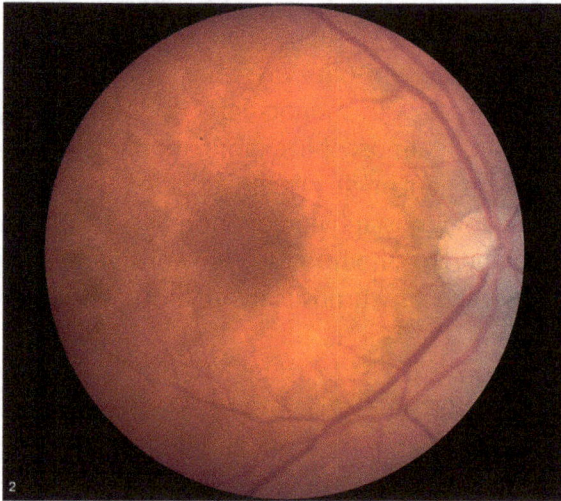

Fig. 14.2. Color photo of the right fundus.

had difficulty seeing objects and words to the left. Ocular examination showed a visual acuity of 20/20 OD and 20/20 OS. Fundus examination (Figs. 14.2 and 14.3) was normal. An MR angiogram (MRA) showed evidence of a right internal carotid artery dissection (Fig. 14.4).

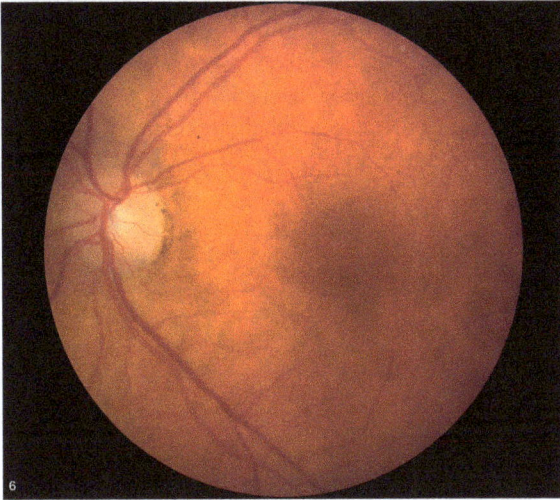

Fig. 14.3. Color photo of the left fundus.

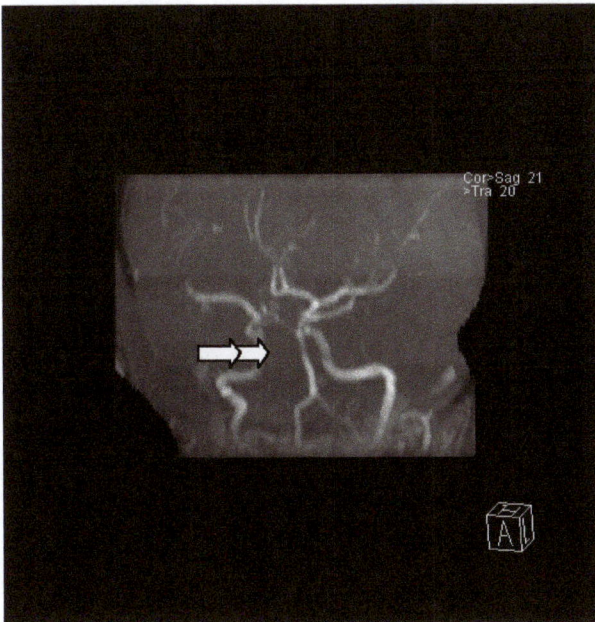

Fig. 14.4. MRA showing a severe narrowing and hypoplastic right internal carotid artery A1 segment suspicious for a carotid artery dissection.

REFERENCES

Biousse V, Touboul PJ, D'Anglejan-Chatillon J, *et al.* (1998) Ophthalmologic manifestations of internal carotid artery dissection. *Am J Ophthalmol* **126**:565–577.
Purvin V, Kawasaki A. (2005) Neuro-ophthalmic emergencies for the neurologist. *Neurologist* **11**:195–233.

15

Jaw Pain and Headache in an Elderly Woman

CASE NO. 15

A 70-year-old woman presents with a three-week history of right sided headache. She described the pain as dull, present throughout the day with no relieving factors. She also admitted to feeling unusually tired and had had an unplanned 10 lb weight loss over the past one month. Over the previous few days, she described pain over the right jaw after chewing her food. She denied any visual symptoms. At a party the previous day, several friends commented on a prominent "bump" which had appeared on the right side of her head (Fig. 15.1). Her husband reported that she was reluctant to comb her hair due to the pain.

Her past medical history was significant for hypertension and osteoarthritis. Regular medication included metoprolol and ibuprofen. There was no family history of headaches. She was a non smoker and did not consume alcohol.

On examination, her visual acuity was 20/25 OD and 20/30 OS. There was no relative afferent pupillary defect. Fundus examination showed possible mild disc pallor OU and the Goldmann perimetry showed mild constriction. An OCT showed normal retinal nerve fiber layer OU. The remainder of the eye exam was normal.

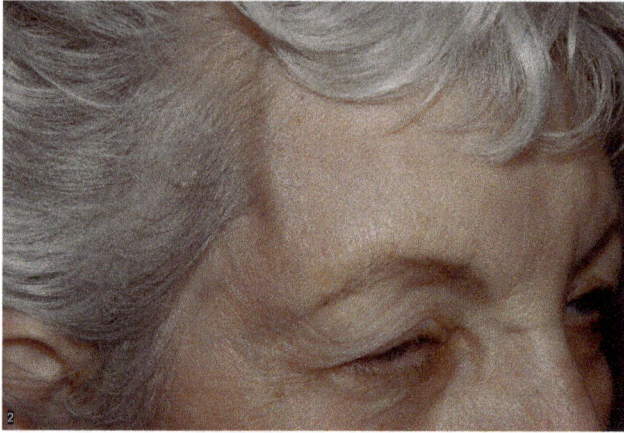

Fig. 15.1. Prominent vessel on the right side of the head.

Dr. Lee. Elderly patients who present with an acute onset of any of the following symptoms or signs should be considered as having giant cell arteritis until proven otherwise:

- new onset headache
- jaw pain or fatigue with chewing
- neck or ear pain
- acute loss of vision
- transient visual loss
- bulging, tender temporal artery
- optic disc edema
- transient diplopia
- unexplained ophthalmoplegia.

Pain when combing the hair or tenderness along the temporal artery is highly suggestive of symptoms of temporal arteritis. A relatively normal eye exam should not dissuade the clinician from consideration of the diagnosis. The most common error for the ophthalmologist would be finding a normal eye exam and then either ignoring or misdiagnosing the headache and other constitutional symptoms. Patients with temporal arteritis may have a prior history of active symptoms of polymyalgia rheumatica (proximal muscle pain in the hip and shoulder girdle with morning stiffness). In patients suspected of having temporal arteritis, I typically start empiric steroids and order both a serum erythrocyte sedimentation rate (ESR) and a C-reactive protein (CRP). Other acute phase reactants (e.g. elevated platelet count) could be considered but I favor the ESR and CRP as screening tests, followed by a unilateral temporal artery biopsy. If the clinical suspicion is high for the diagnosis, I would proceed to a contralateral temporal artery biopsy if the initial biopsy was negative. I tend to treat with prednisone (1.0 to 1.5 mg per kg per day) during the evaluation phase. Although the evidence is somewhat controversial, I do consider intravenous steroids for patients who are monocular, have bilateral simultaneous or rapidly sequential visual symptoms or signs, have severe visual loss (especially if less than a few days of onset), or who have transient visual loss. There is no prospective, randomized, head to head data comparing intravenous to oral steroids, however. Most of my patients with biopsy proven temporal arteritis require therapy for months to years. I write (or call) the primary care doctor to provide them with information about the diagnosis, warn them about the impending steroid related side effects (especially in frail older patients), encourage them not to taper the steroids, and ask them to follow the patient and provide treatment for osteoporosis prophylaxis (e.g. vitamin D, calcium, DEXA bone density).

Dr. Brazis. I agree with Dr. Lee's comments. In our Clinic, we perform a temporal artery biopsy unilaterally and interpret this immediately via frozen section. If the unilateral biopsy is negative, we go on to perform a biopsy on the contralateral side. If the surgeon does not have the "luxury" of frozen section interpretation, I would suggest bilateral biopsies in most patients as the yield of doing the second side is perhaps 2 to 3%, and one never wants to miss this diagnosis because of the potentially catastrophic visual loss that may result if the diagnosis is missed and treatment is not continued. We also suggest intravenous corticosteroids in the scenarios described by Dr Lee. We place all patients on aspirin, if there are no contraindications, as this agent may decrease subsequent ischemic risk; the evidence for the use of aspirin in GCA is anecdotal but might reduce the risk for future cardiovascular events or complications.

Course. Blood results were significant for an ESR of 16 mm/hr and a CRP 2.8 mg/dl (<1.5 normal). The patient was started on oral prednisone 100 mg per day. A temporal artery biopsy was performed despite the normal ESR and showed granulomatous arteritis on the biopsy. The patient was slowly tapered down on the prednisone over an 18-month duration and did not suffer any visual loss or other complications of therapy.

REFERENCES

Lee AG, Brazis PW. (2006) Case studies in neuro-ophthalmology for the neurologist. *Neurol Clin* **24**:331–345.

Lee AG, Brazis PW. (1999) Temporal arteritis: A clinical approach. *J Am Geriatr Soc* **47**:1364–1370.

16

Acute Bitemporal Hemianopsia

CASE NO. 16

A 56-year-old previously healthy man had been a passenger in a car driven by his son when he suddenly complained of headache, blurred vision and feeling dizzy. Shortly after this complaint, he lost consciousness and his son drove him directly to the Emergency Room. His level of consciousness improved and he was brought to the Neuro-Ophthalmology Clinic for further evaluation. On examination, his visual acuity was 20/80 OD and 20/60 OS. There was no relative afferent pupillary defect. Fundus examination showed normal discs (Figs. 16.1, 16.2). The initial consulting ophthalmologist had seen the patient and recommended that he be sent to the eye clinic when stable for a formal visual field. At the bedside, however, the neuro-ophthalmologist performed confrontation testing that suggested a bitemporal hemianopia. Three weeks later a formal Goldmann perimetry, however, confirmed the bitemporal hemianopsia.

Dr. Lee. The acute onset of headache and a bitemporal hemianopia implicates a lesion at the level of the optic chiasm. The life-threatening etiologies for an acute chiasmal syndrome include suprasellar aneurysm and pituitary apoplexy. Chiasmal neuritis could produce the visual field defect and pain but the loss of consciousness suggests a rapidly expanding lesion. Pituitary apoplexy is an emergency because of the associated panhypopituitarism and potentially life-threatening cortisol deficiency which might require emergent admission and hormone replacement. Surgical decompression might

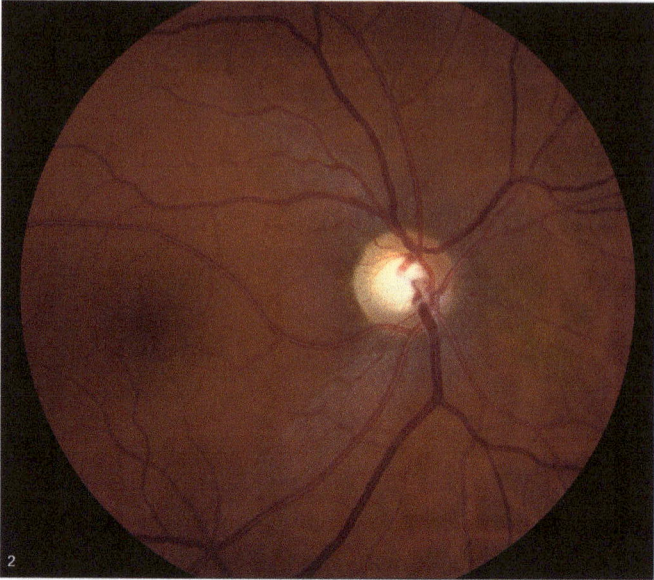

Fig. 16.1. Color picture of the right fundus.

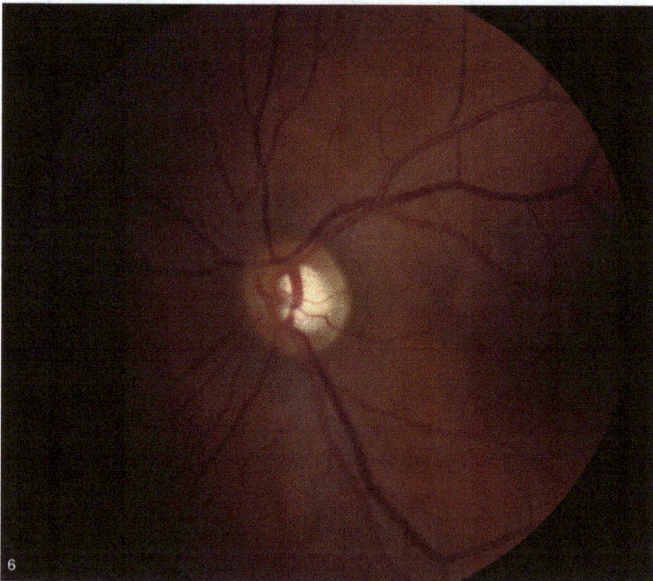

Fig. 16.2. Color picture of the left fundus.

be urgently required as well for a rapidly expanding lesion producing other neurologic deficit (e.g. loss of consciousness as in this case). Although an MRI is generally superior to a CT scan for sellar lesions, a CT scan is faster to obtain and might show hemorrhage from apoplexy that might allow earlier diagnosis and treatment for the patient. The important points for the ophthalmologist are that an acute painful bitemporal hemianopia should be imaged emergently even if the imaging is to be done after working hours or over the weekend and that patients with apoplexy need admission and evaluation for panhypopituitarism and other endocrine dysfunction. The key for the ophthalmologist seeing a patient at the bedside is to perform a confrontation visual field to confirm that the visual field defect is bitemporal and thus localizing. Waiting for the patient to have a formal perimetry out of convenience or delaying the diagnosis while waiting for the patient to be stable enough for transportation to the clinic is not recommended.

Dr Brazis. We warn all patients known to have a pituitary tumor about the possibility of pituitary apoplexy, i.e. sudden expansion of the tumor by ischemia or hemorrhage, and document this warning in the patient's chart. Patients with known pituitary tumors are instructed go to the emergency room immediately if they suffer any sudden, excruciating headache, sudden visual loss, or sudden diplopia. Emergency hormonal replacement and neurosurgical procedure may be live saving.

Course. Cranial CT and MR scans showed a pituitary mass with hemorrhagic components (Figs. 16.3 to 16.7). His son reported in retrospect that the patient had been seen in follow up for a benign "brain tumor" in the past but the surgeons had told him that it did not need surgery yet and his last cranial MRI performed two months ago showed no change. A CT scan in the ER showed a pituitary mass with areas of high density suspicious for a bleed (Figs. 16.3, 16.4).

The patient underwent trans-sphenoidal decompression of his pituitary tumor with secondary apoplexy and recovered completely.

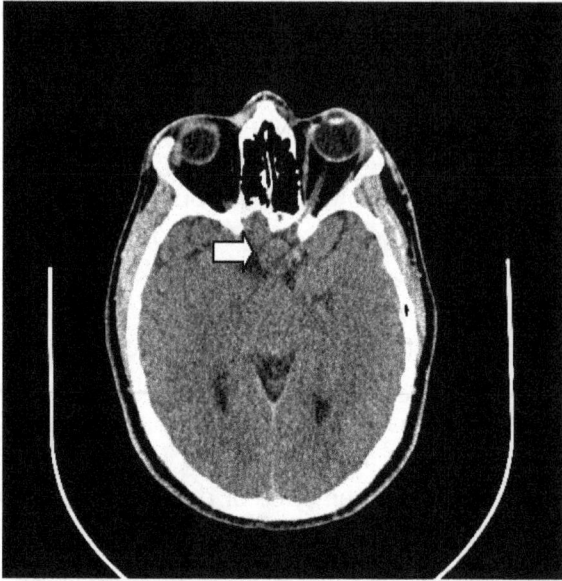

Fig. 16.3. Non contrast CT head showing a mass labeled with an *arrow*.

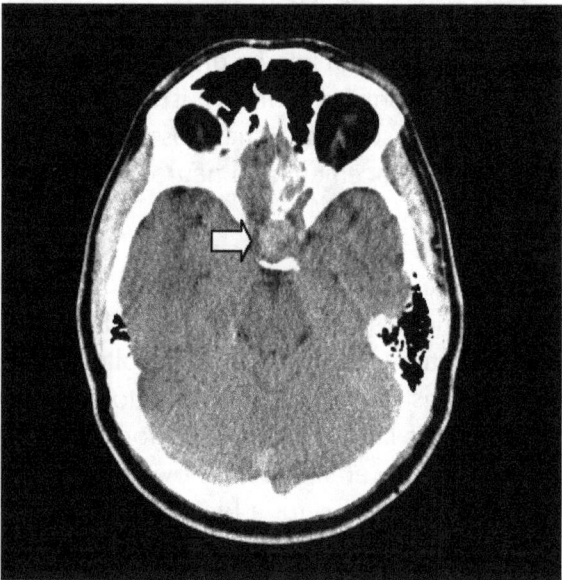

Fig. 16.4. CT head showing areas of high density and low density within the mass.

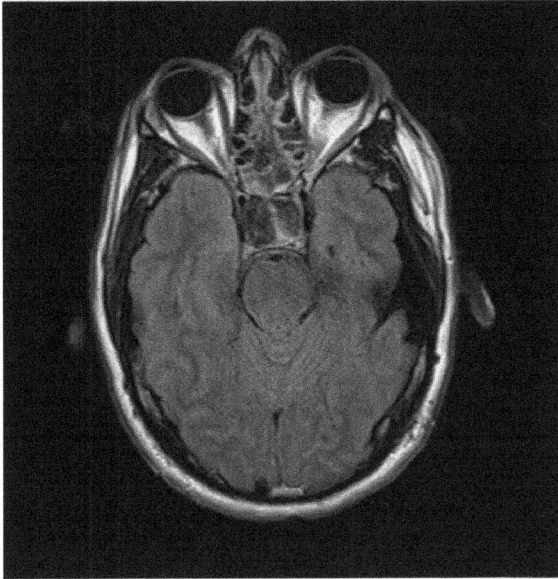

Fig. 16.5. Axial FLAIR MRI showing a large mass with areas of high and low signal within the sella consistent with a pituitary lesion.

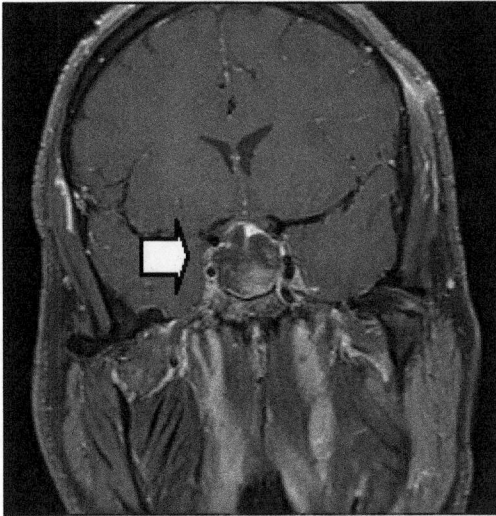

Fig. 16.6. Saggital MRI showing a large mass with rim enhancement and areas of high and low signal within suspicious for hemorrhage.

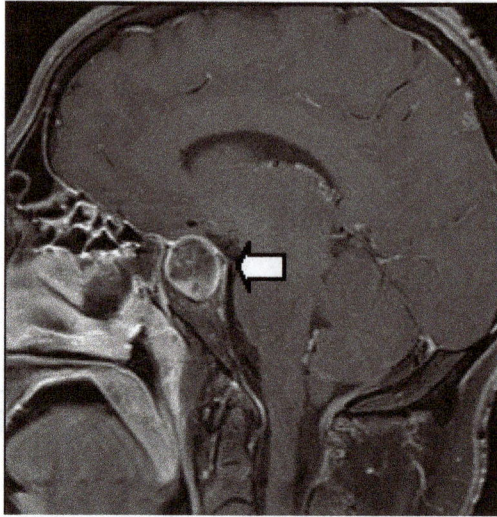

Fig. 16.7. Coronal MRI showing a large mass with rim enhancement and areas of high and low signal within suspicious for hemorrhage.

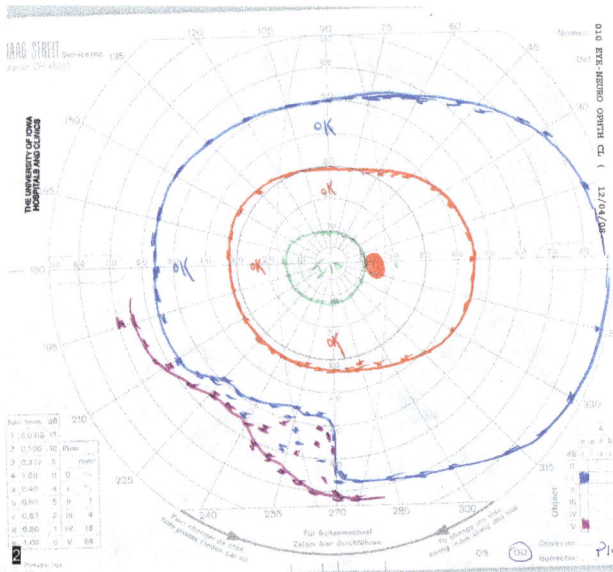

Fig. 16.8. Goldmann perimetry of the right eye showing some inferonasal depression.

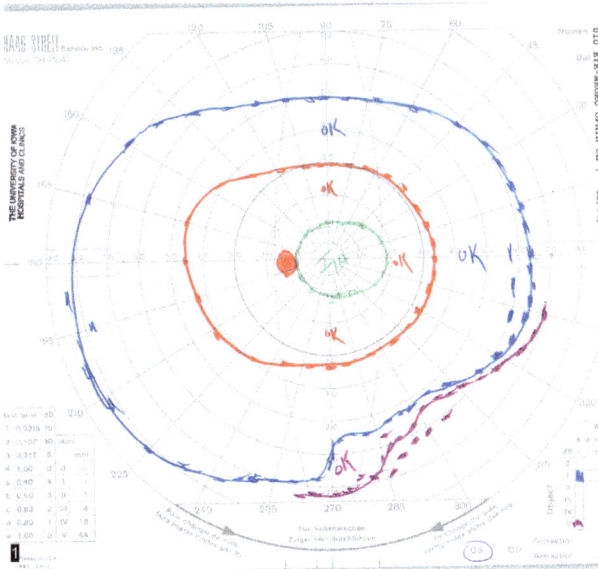

Fig. 16.9. Goldmann perimetry of the left eye showing some inferonasal depression.

Follow-up Goldmann visual fields showed some residual visual field depression but resolution of the prior bitemporal hemianopsia (Figs. 16.8, 16.9).

REFERENCES

da Motta LA, de Mello PA, de Lacerda CM, *et al.* (1999) Pituitary apoplexy. Clinical course, endocrine evaluations and treatment analysis. *J Neurosurg Sci* **43**:25–36.

David NJ. (2006) Pituitary apoplexy goes to the bar: Litigation for delayed diagnosis, deficient vision, and death. *J Neuroophthalmol* **26**:128–133.

Lee AG, Brazis PW. (2006) Case studies in neuro-ophthalmology for the neurologist. *Neurol Clin* **24**:331–345.

17

Acute Anisocoria with Neck Pain

CASE NO. 17

A 54-year-old woman underwent chiropractic treatment for neck pain, and a few days after the neck manipulation, noticed her right lid started drooping. Her husband noticed that the right pupil was significantly smaller than the left. She denied any vision loss or diplopia. The patient reported worsening of her right-sided neck pain and she was referred to the neuro-ophthalmology service. Past family history was significant for diabetes and hypertension. She did not smoke cigarettes or consume alcohol. She was allergic to penicillin and did not take any medication. The remainder of the medical history was non-contributory.

On examination, her visual acuity was 20/20 OU. The right pupil was miotic and measured 3 mm in the dark and 2 mm in the light with no afferent pupillary defect. The light and near reaction are normal in each pupil. The left pupil measured 4 mm in the dark and 2.5 mm in the light (Fig. 17.1). There was a 1 mm right ptosis and minimal "upside down ptosis" OD. A dilation lag was demonstrated OD clinically with the anisocoria greater at 5 seconds in dim ambient light as compared to 15 seconds. The remainder of the ocular and neurologic exam was normal.

Discussion

Dr. Lee. The comprehensive ophthalmologist confronted with acute neck pain and anisocoria should first determine if the big pupil or the small pupil is the problem. The "big pupil" problem associated with

155

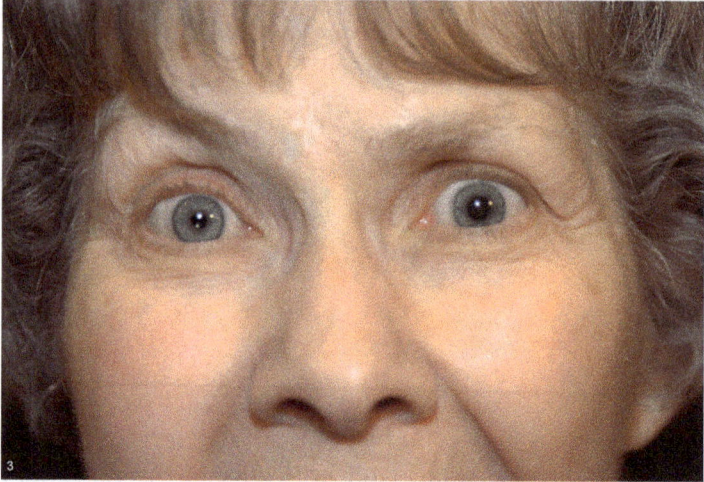

Fig. 17.1. External photograph showing anisocoria with the right pupil smaller than the left in the light.

pain is the pupil-involved third nerve palsy. The "small pupil" emergency is the Horner syndrome. Patients with a Horner syndrome may be harboring a lesion anywhere along the ocular sympathetic pathway from the hypothalamus, down the brainstem to the thoracic cord (C8-T2 level), up the sympathetic chain in the neck, to the internal carotid artery, the cavernous sinus, and finally the ipsilateral orbit. In the acute setting with pain, the major life-threatening etiology for a Horner syndrome is an ipsilateral internal carotid artery dissection. In this case, the right pupil is miotic and the papillary light and near reactions are otherwise normal in each eye. The anisocoria is greater in the dark than in the light. This implicates the small pupil as the abnormal pupil. In the setting of mild ptosis or upside down ptosis, this anisocoria is a Horner syndrome until proven otherwise. The dilation lag is confirmatory evidence for a Horner syndrome. The major differential diagnosis for the anisocoria would include physiologic anisocoria but the constellation of findings in this patient suggests a Horner syndrome. In the acute setting with convincing clinical findings I would recommend performing a same day MRI study of the oculosympathetic pathway from the hypothalamus (i.e. cranial MRI) to the T2 level in the chest with particular attention to the ipsilateral internal carotid artery to exclude dissection. The history of chiropractic manipulation is suggestive of a potential mechanism for a carotid dissection. The evidence for the role of chiropractic manipulation is controversial but anecdotal evidence suggests a possible causal relationship. Unfortunately, many patients are visiting the chiropractor because of neck pain and perhaps these patients had pre-existing Horner syndrome that is coincidentally linked to the chiropractic manipulation and not necessarily causally linked. Topical cocaine has been the traditional pharmacologic test for distinguishing the Horner syndrome from physiologic anisocoria. Topical cocaine has become more and more difficult for comprehensive ophthalmologists to obtain and keep on hand in compliance with hospital, state, and federal regulatory policies and procedures. A topical cocaine test is generally considered positive if the post-drop anisocoria is 0.8 mm or greater. A follow-up hydroxyamphetamine test can localize the lesion to pre- or post-ganglionic location. Cocaine inhibits the re-uptake of norepinephrine at the junction and a positive cocaine test confirms a Horner syndrome. In contrast, hydroxyamphetamine stimulates the release of norepinephrine at the junction and thus can distinguish a pre- from post-ganglionic Horner syndrome. Recently, we have been using topical apraclonidine for our Horner syndrome testing. Apraclonidine demonstrates a differential alpha-1 and alpha-2 effects on normal and Horner syndrome pupils. In patients with a Horner syndrome, topical apraclonidine will reverse the anisocoria with the larger pupil becoming smaller and the smaller pupil becoming larger. This endpoint is easier to detect and interpret than the post-drop anisocoria measurements for the topical cocaine test. In the acute setting, however, especially with neck pain the clinician does not have time to perform these confirmatory and localizing pharmacologic tests and it has been our practice to simply proceed to emergent imaging of the entire oculosympathetic pathway with a single MRI study of the head and neck with or without a concomitant MR angiogram (MRA) to exclude dissection. The distinctive radiographic sign of the carotid dissection is a crescent of high signal intensity on T1 that represents the dissected segment and blood. Patients with an acute internal carotid artery dissection should probably be evaluated by the neurologist and considered for admission, further evaluation, and antiplatelet treatment. The role of anticoagulation (e.g. warfarin) versus antiplatelet treatment remains controversial and this decision is best left to the admitting and treating neurologist. The main role of the ophthalmologist is to identify the Horner syndrome and order the appropriate neuroimaging study including the neck. The most common error that the ophthalmologist can make in the evaluation of the Horner syndrome is imaging the head only and forgetting about the extracranial components of the oculosympathetic pathway. The major potential life-threatening etiologies for the Horner syndrome are the internal carotid dissection in the neck and a tumor in the lung apex (i.e. the Pancoast tumor) which would be missed if only the brain was imaged. The second most common neuroimaging error would be to order a computed tomography (CT) scan alone as the MRI is more sensitive for the detection of the extracranial carotid dissection than the CT scan. The third most common diagnostic error is not realizing the urgency of evaluation for an acute Horner syndrome as patients with an internal carotid dissection might suffer an ipsilateral hemispheric stroke from thromboembolic disease or have a potentially treatable dissection that requires emergent evaluation. The bottom line is that for this patient with an acute painful Horner syndrome after chiropractic manipulation of the neck, I would recommend an MRI and MRA of the head and neck to rule out extracranial internal carotid artery dissection. If apraclonidine or topical cocaine drops are available, it might be of interest to confirm the clinical suspicion but if they are unavailable or if pharmacologic testing would delay the imaging, then I would just proceeding to the neuroimaging study recommended above.

Dr. Brazis. A Horner syndrome may be caused by a lesion anywhere along the sympathetic pathway that supplies the head, eye, and neck. Associated symptoms and signs usually allow localization of the lesion.

When you see a patient with new anisocoria possibly related to a Horner syndrome, you should confirm the presence of a Horner syndrome pharmacologically (with cocaine or apraclonidine). The evaluation of an adult with Horner syndrome is mostly based on lesion location. The most classic cause of central (first order neuron) Horner is a lateral medullary infarction (Wallenberg syndrome); other causes include various thalamic, brainstem, and spinal cord lesions. Second-order Horner syndromes are most suggestive of neoplasm or trauma of the lower cervical spine, brachial plexus, or lung apex. Third-order Horner syndromes point to lesions of the internal carotid artery such as dissection or cavernous sinus aneurysms. Further evaluation depends on the duration of symptoms, the presence of pain, other symptoms or signs, and the localization of the lesion to the 1st/2nd order neuron or to the 3rd order neuron.

All patients need a physical examination (ocular, neurologic, neck, supraclavicular, and chest). The tests ordered will vary depending on the lesion location, the presence of associated symptoms or signs, the urgency of the work-up, and the radiologists' preference. If a 1st or 2nd order Horner is present, we suggest a CT or MRI of the chest (to view pulmonary apex), MRI of head and neck with contrast, and possibly an MRA of the aortic arch or CTA (CT angiogram) of the head and neck. If a 3rd order Horner is present, we suggest MRI of the head with contrast and MRA or CTA of the head and neck. If localization of the Horner syndrome is unknown, we suggest imaging the brain, neck, spinal cord, carotid arteries, and pulmonary apex (may require multiple imaging tests). We feel that in this situation the easiest test is MRI and MRA of the head, neck, and pulmonary apex using pre-defined Horner protocols. Some authorities suggest a CT/CTA of the head, neck, and chest, which allows good examination of the brain and spine, the soft tissues, and large blood vessels in the head, neck and chest; it also allows examination of the pulmonary apex.

An acute painful Horner syndrome should be presumed related to a dissection of the ipsilateral internal carotid artery unless proven otherwise. These patients are at risk for cerebral infarction and should be evaluated emergently.

Course. External photographs were taken before (Fig. 17.2) and after pharmacologic testing. Note that the topical cocaine has eliminated

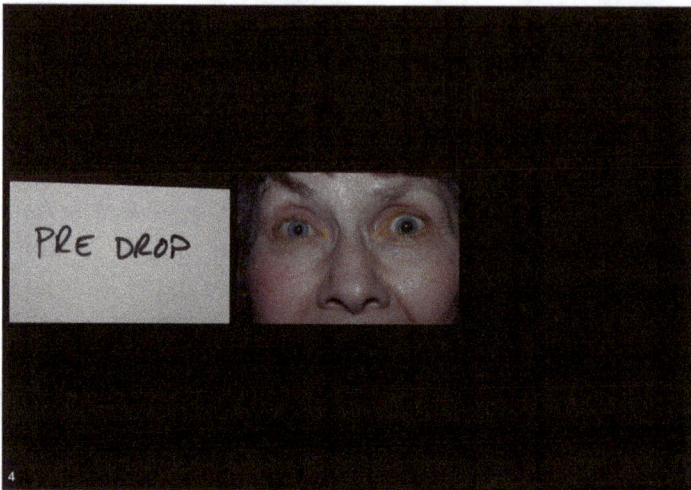

Fig. 17.2. External appearance prior to instillation of cocaine drops.

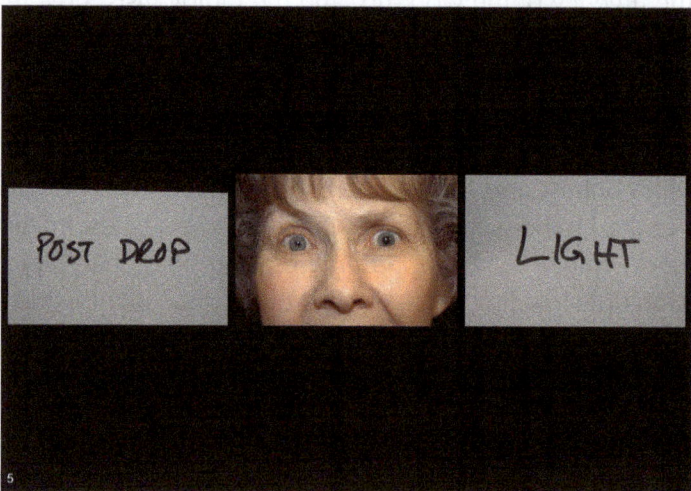

Fig. 17.3. External appearance following the administration of cocaine drops in the light.

the pre-drop test ptosis in the post-drop photos. Topical cocaine administration confirmed a right Horner's syndrome (Figs. 17.3 to 17.4) with a residual anisocoria of greater than 1 mm after the topical testing. Magnetic resonance (MR) imaging of the neck

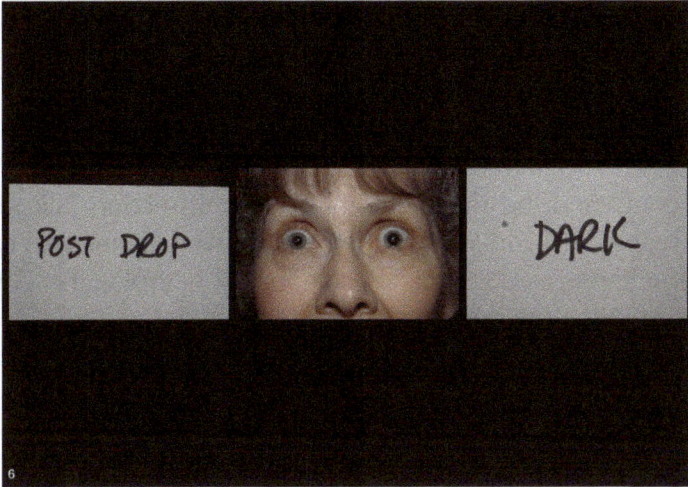

Fig. 17.4. External appearance following cocaine administration in the dark.

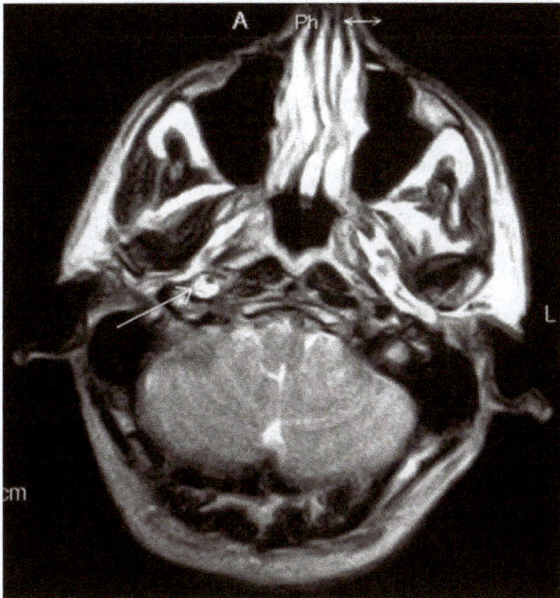

Fig. 17.5. MRI with gadolinium contrast showing right internal carotid artery dissection labeled with an *arrow*. The "crescent sign" of hyperintense T1 signal surrounding the dark circular flow void of the right internal carotid artery (*black circle*).

showed a crescent sign of high intensity on the T1 surrounding the right internal carotid artery, consistent with a carotid dissection (Fig. 17.5). Following the MRI, the patient was admitted to the hospital and treated with antiplatelet therapy with aspirin. The brain MRI showed no intracranial ischemia. The neck MR angiogram (MRA) confirmed the right internal carotid dissection. Six months later, a repeat MRI and MRA of the neck showed the internal carotid dissection had healed completely. No further neurologic events had developed in the interim.

REFERENCES

Biousse V, Touboul PJ, D'Anglejan-Chatillon J, *et al.* (1998) Ophthalmologic manifestations of internal carotid artery dissection. *Am J Ophthalmol* **126**:565–577.

Cremer SA, Thompson HS, Digre KB, Kardon RH. (1990) Hydroxyamphetamine mydriasis in Horner's syndrome. *Am J Ophthalmol* **110**:71–6.2368824.

Freedman KA, Brown SM. (2005) Topical apraclonidine in the diagnosis of suspected Horner syndrome. *J Neuroophthalmol* **25**:83–85.

Kardon RH, Denison CE, Brown CK, Thompson HS. (1990) Critical evaluation of the cocaine test in the diagnosis of Horner's syndrome. *Arch Ophthalmol* **108**:384–387.

Reede DL, Garcon E, Smoker WR, Kardon R. (2008) Horner's syndrome: Clinical and radiographic evaluation. *Neuroimaging Clin N Am* **18**:369–385.

18

Acute Painful Ophthalmoplegia

CASE NO. 18

A 37-year-old African American female presented with an acute onset of painful ophthalmoplegia OS. Her past medical, family, surgical, and social history were unremarkable. She was taking no medications. She did not smoke or consume alcohol. She had no other neurologic signs or symptoms.

Exam

The patient's visual acuity was 20/20 OU. The pupils were 4 mm OU and were reactive to light bilaterally. There was no relative afferent pupillary defect. The motility exam showed a primary position exotropia of 40 prism diopters that increased on gaze to the left to >55 prism diopters. There was limitation of adduction, elevation, and depression OD and there was a mild abduction deficit OD as well (Fig. 18.1). Her pain was limited to the V1 distribution on the face OD and she had mildly decreased cutaneous pinprick sensation in the V1 distribution on the right. The fourth nerve function seemed intact with intorsion in downgaze seen OD.

Dr. Brazis. In a patient with ophthalmoplegia and ophthalmic branch trigeminal (V1) distribution pain or numbness, a cavernous sinus lesion should be considered. The mild abduction deficit is also suggestive of a partial sixth nerve dysfunction. Combined ocular motor paresis and sympathetic denervation (not seen in this patient) are virtually pathognomonic of a cavernous sinus lesion. Compressive

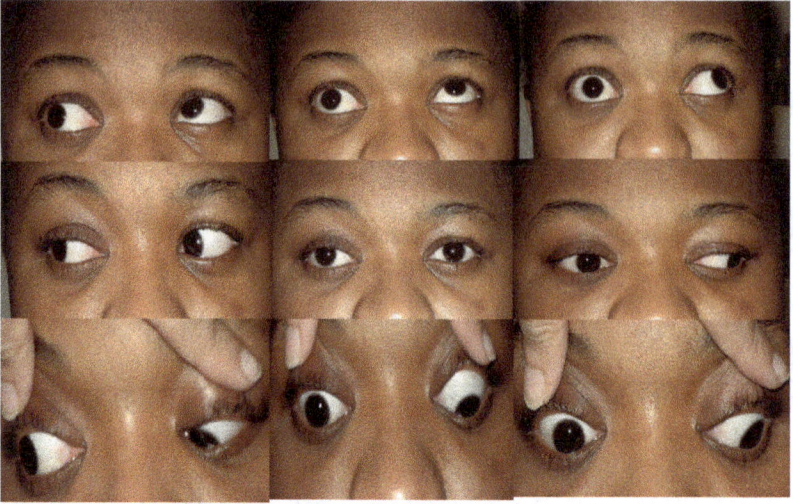

Fig. 18.1. Motility photographs show the limitation of elevation, depression and adduction OD. There was a minimal abduction deficit OD as well with a small esotropia in right gaze of 5 prism diopters. Note that the primary position deviation is not as large as one might expect from a medial rectus palsy alone, suggesting that the mild abduction deficit OD is an associated sixth nerve palsy.

cavernous sinus lesions may also spare the pupil because they often preferentially involve only the superior division of the oculomotor nerve, which carries no pupillomotor fibers, or the superior aspect of the nerve anterior to the point where the pupillomotor fibers descend in their course near the inferior oblique muscle. The pupillary "sparing" with anterior cavernous sinus lesions may be more apparent than real, resulting from simultaneous injury of nerve fibers to both the pupillary sphincter and dilator, resulting in a midposition, fixed pupil. The sympathetic fibers to the eye join the abducens nerve for a short distance within the cavernous sinus, and thus a unilateral abducens nerve lesion associated with an ipsilateral Horner syndrome is of localizing value.

Pituitary adenomas, nasopharyngeal carcinomas, craniopharyngiomas, and metastases most commonly may cause a cavernous sinus syndrome. Sphenoid sinus carcinoma often causes a spheno-cavernous syndrome, but may also present with an isolated sixth nerve palsy. Nasopharyngeal carcinoma may compress the sixth nerve as many of these tumors arise from the fossa of Rosenmuller immediately beneath the foramen lacerum. Extension of the tumor through the foramen lacerum may cause a trigeminal sensory loss (e.g. affecting a V2 distribution) and a sixth nerve palsy. Thus, the combination of facial pain or V2 sensory loss with a sixth nerve palsy is a common presentation of nasopharyngeal carcinoma. Serous otitis media is a frequent accompaniment due to blockage of the Eustacian tube.

Carotid-cavernous sinus dural arteriovenous fistulae may present with unilateral or bilateral cavernous sinus syndromes. Tolosa–Hunt syndrome, which is caused by inflammatory processes of various etiologies involving the cavernous sinus, presents with ocular motor weakness and retroorbital pain. Facial sensation and visual acuity may be diminished. Tolosa–Hunt syndrome or painful ophthalmo-plegia is a diagnosis of exclusion. Sudden onset of headache and dysfunction of multiple ocular motor nerves on either one or both sides, with or without retroorbital pain or visual impairment, suggests the possibility of pituitary apoplexy. In all patients with a cavernous sinus syndrome, infectious etiologies, especially due to *Aspergillus* or Mucormycosis, are of concern, especially if the patient is immuno-compromised.

The patient described needs an MRI with specific attention to the cavernous sinus and superior orbital fissure regions.

Dr. Lee. I completely agree with Dr. Brazis that the combination of an ispilateral third, fifth (V1), and in this case a possible sixth nerve palsy suggests a cavernous sinus localization. The Tolosa–Hunt syndrome is a painful ophthalmoplegia syndrome that is typically steroid responsive and is as Dr. Brazis said, a "diagnosis of exclu-sion." I generally order an MRI with contrast and I direct specific attention to the ipsilateral cavernous sinus. The International Headache Society (IHS) redefined the prior diagnostic criteria for the entity known as the "Tolosa–Hunt syndrome" (THS). The diagnostic criteria require that granuloma be demonstrated by MRI or biopsy. La Mantia *et al.* reviewed the literature on THS from 1988 to 2002 and found 124 THS cases. Forty-four cases (35%) had inflammation on MRI or biopsy, evidence of granuloma, and 41/124 (33%) had normal neuroimaging. Interestingly, 39 (31%) had a specific cause and so the THS was "secondary." The authors concluded that the clinical presentations for THS are common to several conditions and "their application alone does not guarantee a correct diagnosis."

Most of the cases of THS referred to me end up being secondary to an underlying and potentially treatable etiology and I would caution the readers to use the diagnosis with caution.

Course. This patient underwent a contrast MRI (Fig. 18.2) which showed enhancement in the right cavernous sinus. An extensive

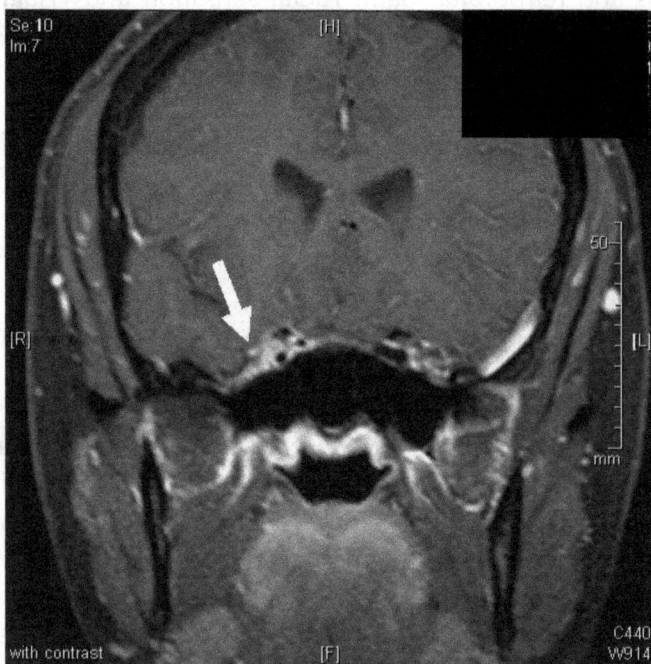

Fig. 18.2. Coronal MRI with contrast shows posterior cavernous sinus enhancement (*arrow*).

evaluation for alternative etiologies was performed and was negative, and a presumptive diagnosis of the Tolosa–Hunt syndrome was made. Intravenous steroid therapy alleviated the patient's pain. In patients with a negative radiographic and laboratory evaluation, complete resolution of clinical signs and symptoms and radiographic findings, and no recurrence of findings after steroid treatment, the diagnosis of Tolosa–Hunt syndrome can be presumed without necessarily pursuing a biopsy.

Index

A

abducens nerve, 53, 164
abscesses, 45–49
acalculia, 44
acetazolamide, 32, 39, 42
acetominophen, 33
activated protein C resistance, 28
Addison's disease, 29
Adie tonic pupil, 122–124
age of patients
  carotid-cavernous sinus fistulae
    and, 3
  leukemia and, 109
  ODEMS and, 128, 129
  optic neuritis and, 65–68
  tissue plasminogen activator
    (tPA) treatment and, 16
  vasculopathic risk factors, 84,
    134
agnosia, finger, 44
alcohol consumption, 115, 117
alexia, 44
all-trans-retinoic acid (ATRA), 29

amaurosis fugax, 133–142
anemia, 113
aneurysms
  central nervous system
    impairment, 45
  cranial nerve palsies and, 55, 56,
    80, 82–87
  giant basilar artery tip, 61
  internal carotid artery, 6, 89
  intracavernous carotid, 5, 6, 55,
    82, 159
  middle cerebral artery (MCA),
    91, **92**, 94
  ophthalmic artery, 69, 74
  posterior communicating artery,
    86, 89, 91, **92**, 94
  signs and symptoms, 123
  suprasellar, 147
angioplasty, 19, 29
anisocoria, 9, 21, 81, 115, 117,
  121–125, 155–162
anorexia, 117
anosognosia, 44

Page numbers in bold type indicate figures.

anterior chamber, 1, 139
antibiotics, 130
anticoagulants, 17, 29, 158
antiphospholipid antibody
    syndrome, 28
antiplatelet therapy, 23, 158, 162
antithrombin III deficiency, 28
aortic vascular disease, 138
aphasia, 44, 134
applanation tonometry, 4, 11
apraclonidine test, topical,
    157–159
apraxia, 44
arteriovenous malformations
    (AVM), 26, 29
aspirin, 145, 146, 162
ataxia, 54, 109, 116, 117
atrial fibrillation, 19
atropine, 124
autotopagnosia, 44

B

bacteria, abscess-causing, 45, 46
Balint syndrome, 61
balloons, detachable, 7
barbiturates, 61
bariatric surgery, 115, 116. *See
    also* obesity
Bartter's syndrome, 29
basilar artery, 61, **62**
behavioral changes, 59, 61. *See
    also* mental status changes
Behçet disease, 28, 29
Bell's phenomenon, 59
Bickerstaff's encephalitis, 62
bipolar disorder, 115

blepharoplasty, 104
blood glucose, 17, 55
blood tests, 17, 26, 48, 55, 117,
    146
botulism, 62
brainstem conditions, 52, 54, 56,
    79, 116, 156
breast cancer, 100
bruit, 1, 4, 9, 12. *See also* tinnitus,
    pulse-synchronous

C

calcium channel blockers, 139
cancer. *See* tumors
carbamazepine, 61
cardiac disease, 17, 134, 135, 138
carotid arterial system, 2, 3. *See
    also* internal carotid artery
carotid-cavernous sinus fistula
    (CCF), 1–8, 9–13, 165
carotid occlusive disease, 136,
    138, 139
cataracts, 137, 139
catheter angiography
    in carotid-cavernous sinus
        fistulae, 5, 6, 11
    in strokes, 22–23
    in third nerve palsies, 83–87,
        89–91
cat scratch disease, 127–131
cavernous sinus
    aneurysms, 55
    carotid arterial system and, 2, 3
    enlargement, 6
    flow voids, 6, 11
    Horner syndrome and, 156

hypotropia, 9
hypoxia, 60

I

iatrogenic conditions, 3, 28, 45,
    55, 115, 116, 138
ibuprofen, 33, 143
idiopathic intracranial
    hypertension (IIH). *See*
    pseudotumor cerebri (PTC)
immunodeficient patients, 46, 113
immunotherapy, 112
indomethacin, 29
infection, 4, 28, 43–49, 67, 113,
    129
inflammatory disease, 28, 101
interferon beta-1a, 71, 72
internal carotid artery
    in carotid-cavernous sinus
        fistulae, 2–4, 8, 11
    Horner syndrome and, 156, 158,
        159, **161**, 162
    third nerve palsies and, 89
    transient visual loss and, 139, 140
International Headache Society
    (IHS), 165, 166
intracerebral and -cranial
    abscesses, 45, 46–49
intracranial pressure (ICP), 6, 26,
    28, 37, 60, 111
intracranial shunting procedure, 39
intracranial vessels, 6, 26, 27, 40
intraocular pressure (IOP)
    with anisocoria, 122
    in carotid-cavernous sinus
        fistula, 1, 5, 9, 11

in early multiple sclerosis, 65
management, 11
in optic neuritis, 65
in pseudotumor cerebri, 25
in third nerve palsies, 77
in thyroid eye disease, 98
iris trauma, 122–124
isotretinoin, 29

J

jaw claudication, 15, 54, 84
jugular veins, 28

K

Kepone, 29
ketaprofen, 29

L

lacrimation, 98, 100
La Mantia, L, 166
Lasix, 77
Leber's idiopathic stellate
    neuroretinitis, 128
Leber's stellate maculopathy, 127
leptomeningeal carcinomatosis, 82
leukemia, 109–113
leukocytosis, 48, 49
lid
    Cogan's lid twitch sign, 52, 79
    Collier's "tucked lid" sign, 60, 61
    edema, 9, 12, 52, 79, 98
    margin repositioning surgery,
        104
    retraction, 97, 99, 101, 104,
        106, 124
lipid maculopathy, 66

when combing hair, 143
pamidronate, 101
panhypopituitarism, 147, 149
panuveitis, 137
papilledema
  etiologies, 27, 29
  management, 26, 27, 29–30, 32, 39
  in pseudotumor cerebri, 26, 39
  signs and symptoms, 36, 37, 40
  sixth nerve palsies and, 56
  typical profile, 39
  use of term, 37
  vs leukemic infiltration of optic nerve, 111
  vs ODEMS, 130
parasympathicolytic drugs, 124
parenteral nutrition, 116
parietal lobe lesions, 21, 43, 139
Parkinson's disease, 61
penicillin, 155
peripapillary exudates, 128
peripapillary staphyloma, 138, 139
phenylephrine, 124
photophobia, 89, 98
piercings causing infection, 43–49
pilocarpine, 122–124
pituitary adenoma, 164
pituitary apoplexy, 74, 85, 147–153, 165
pleocytosis, 68
polycythemia vera, 138
polymyalgia rheumatica, 84, 145
posterior cerebral artery, 22, **23**
posterior ciliary artery, 137

posterior communicating artery, 86, 89, 91, **92**, 94
post-partum patients, 29, 115
prednisone, 70, 145, 146
pregnancy, 27, 29, 40
pretectal syndrome, 60
proptosis
  alternative etiologies, 99
  carotid-cavernous sinus fistula and, 1, 3–6, 9, 12
  cranial nerve palsies and, 54, 79
  exclusionary sign, 52
  Graves' ophthalmopathy and, 98, 102, 104
  orbital myositis and, 100, 102
  surgical decompression, 105
prostate cancer, 101
protein S deficiency, 28
protime (PT), 17
pseudoabducens palsy, 61
pseudoaneurysms, 5
pseudotumor cerebri (PTC), 26–32, 39, 40
psychosocial factors, 40, 70
ptosis
  absence of, 21
  bilateral, 60
  exclusionary sign, 52
  Horner syndrome and, 155, 156, 159–161
  orbital myositis and, 99
  sign of carotid-cavernous sinus fistula, 1, **2**, 9, 12
  with third nerve palsy, 77–79, 87, 89
pulmonary apex, 159

smoking, 81, 103–104, 106, 133, 134, 138
spatial disorientation, 44
spinal cord, 109
spinal tap. *See* lumbar puncture (LP)
statin therapy, 51, 77
stenting, 19, 29
stereopsis, 66
steroids
    ODEMS and, 130
    optic neuropathy and, 67, 70, 106
    orbital myositis and, 99
    pseudotumor cerebri and, 29
    temporal arteritis and, 145
    Tolosa-Hunt syndrome and, 165, 167
strabismus, 99, 104
stroke
    in carotid-cavernous sinus fistula treatment, 8
    etiologies, 19
    homonymous hemianopsia and, 15–20
    Horner syndrome and, 158, 159
    mimic, 19
    risk factors, 134, 138
    signs and symptoms, 15–17, 21, 59–61
    treatment, 16–20, 22, 23, 61–63
subarachnoid hemorrhaging (SAH)
    carotid-cavernous sinus fistula and, 3, 6
    catheter angiography and, 89, 90
    cranial nerve palsies and, 56, 85

CT scanning for, 81, 83
intracranial pressure and, 26
pupil dilation and, 123
tissue plasminogen activator (tPA) and, 17
superior vena cava syndrome, 28
surgical decompression, 104–106, 147–149
syphilis, 61, 68, 130
systemic lupus erythematosus (SLE), 28, 29, 67, 81, 99, 101, 138

T
telemedicine, 19
temporal arteritis, 55, 143–146
temporal artery biopsies, 55, 84, 145, 146
temporal lobe lesions, 21, 61
tetracyclines, 29, 33
thiamine, 116–118
third nerve palsies, 62, 77–87, 89–96, 122–124, 156
thrombocythemia, 28
thromboembolic disease, 22, 135, 139, 158
thrombolytic treatments, 18, 29
thrombosis, 3, 5, 6, 28, 40
thyroid eye disease, 9, 97–106
thyroid replacement, 29
tinnitus, pulse-synchronous, 4, 33, 36
tissue plasminogen activator (tPA), 16–19, 22, 61, 62
Todd's paralysis, 19